Using Alternative Therapies: A Qualitative Analysis

Jacqueline Low

Canadian Scholars' Press Inc.
Toronto

Using Alternative Therapies: A Qualitative Analysis
by Jacqueline Low

First published in 2004 by
Canadian Scholars' Press Inc.
180 Bloor Street West, Suite 801
Toronto, Ontario
M5S 2V6

www.cspi.org

Portions of chapter one, "What Are Alternative Therapies and Who Uses Them?" were originally published in Low, J. (2001), "Alternative, complementary, or concurrent health care? A critical analysis of the use of the concept of complementary therapy," *Complementary Therapies in Medicine*, 9(2):105–110. Reproduced with permission from Harcourt Publishers, Ltd. Portions of the conclusion were previously published in Low, J. (2003), "Lay assessments of the efficacy of alternative/complementary therapies: a challenge to medical and expert dominance?," *Evidence-Based Integrative Medicine*, 1(1):65–76. Reproduced with permission from Open Minds Journals.

Every reasonable effort has been made to identify copyright holders. CSPI would be pleased to have any errors or omissions brought to its attention.

Canadian Scholars' Press gratefully acknowledges financial support for our publishing activities from the Government of Canada through the Book Publishing Industry Development Program (BPIDP) and the Government of Ontario through the Ontario Book Publishing Tax Credit Program.

National Library of Canada Cataloguing in Publication

Low, Jacqueline, 1964–
Using alternative therapies : a qualitative analysis / Jacqueline Low.

Includes bibliographical references and index.
ISBN 1-55130-264-0

I. Alternative medicine--Canada--Case studies. I. Title.

R733.L68 2004   615.5   C2004-900196-5

Cover and text design by Hothouse Canada

04 05 06 07 08   5 4 3 2 1

Printed and bound in Canada by AGMV Marquis Imprimeur Inc.

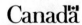

DEDICATION

This book is dedicated, with love, to the memory
of my brother, Douglas, who never failed to encourage me
or tell me of the pride he took in my scholarly achievements.

Table of Contents

Preface

In this book I present a qualitative analysis of the experiences of twenty-one Canadians who use alternative therapies. My analysis is informed by a symbolic interactionist perspective that emphasizes the process by which people give meaning to reality, and how those meanings guide their actions. This research is a timely addition to the literature on alternative and complementary health care as it addresses significant gaps in this area of scholarship. For instance, dominant biomedical interests mean that there is considerable study of the therapies themselves, especially the issues of efficacy and safety (Ernst 1997, 1999, 2000a; Lewith et al. 2000). An equally pervasive concentration on the professions means that research is, more often than not, geared towards the study of the activities of alternative practitioners in their efforts to professionalize or achieve regulated status (Boon 1998; Bourgeault 2000; Coburn 1997; Saks 1995). While the aforementioned are certainly valid research concerns, preoccupation with them turns attention away from the lay person who participates in these approaches to health and healing. Moreover, even when the focus of research is on the user of these therapies, the overwhelming majority of studies employ quantitative methods (Eisenberg et al. 1998; Blais 2000; Furnham 1994; Vincent and Furnham 1994, 1996, 1997). While quantitative approaches can provide us with information about the number of people who use alternative health care, as well as about their broad demographic characteristics, they tell us less about the wider experiences people have with alternative therapies and the impact of those experiences on their lives.

The study of alternative therapy has also been dominated by British and American scholarship. While the last ten years has seen the burgeoning of attention to the study of alternative health and healing by Canadian scholars,[1] little international research has addressed participation in alternative health care in the Canadian context. For instance, in documenting the usage of alternative and complementary therapies in the United Kingdom (UK) and internationally, Fulder (1996:xii) refers to "the United States, Western Europe, Germany, France, The Netherlands, the rest of Europe and Scandinavia, ... Russia and Eastern Europe, Australia, New Zealand, ... South Africa, ... China [and] India"—but makes no mention of the use of alternative therapies in Canada. Therefore, my intent in this book is to address these gaps in the literature by furthering understanding of how and why Canadians seek out alternative health care, of their beliefs about these approaches to health and healing, and of what impact participation in these therapies has on them.

This work will be of particular interest to sociologists and other social scientists researching and teaching in the areas of health and health care, as well as in those of alternative and complementary therapies. It will also be useful for graduate and undergraduate students in health studies programs or those majoring in sociology and social sciences with a focus on health, illness, and health care. Given my attention to issues of identity construction and stigma management, this book can also serve as a supplementary text in courses dealing with such subjects as "the self and identity" as well as "deviant behaviour." In addition, given the increasing interest in integrating alternative and complementary therapies within the Canadian health care system (Tataryn and Verhoef 2001; Balon et al. 2001a), this book will prove useful as reference material for health care professionals and health policymakers. Finally, I hope that this study and its findings will be of interest to those members of the general public who participate in alternative therapies, or who wish to learn more about alternative forms of health and healing.

NOTES

1. See Achilles (2001); Achilles et al. (1999); Anyinam (1990); Balon et al. (2001a, 2001b); Blais (2000); Boon (1998); Boon et al. (1999); Bourgeault (2000); Bourgeault and Fynes (1997); Cain et al (1999); Casey and Picherack (2001); Coburn (1997); Coburn and Biggs (1987); Connor (1997); Coulter (1985); Crellin et al. (1997); de Bruyn (2001); Gort and Coburn (1997); Kelner (2000); Kelner et al. (1986); Kelner and Wellman (2000, 1997); Low (2001a, 2001b, 2003, 2004); Montbriand and Laing (1991); Northcott (1994, 2002); Northcott and Bachynsky (1993); Pawluch et al. (1994, 1998a, 1998b); Ramsay et al. (1999); Sévigny et al. (1990); and Tataryn and Verhoef (2001).

Acknowledgements

I am grateful to William Shaffir, Dorothy Pawluch, and Roy Cain, who supervised the dissertation research from which this book emerged. Professor Shaffir's expertise in qualitative methods and symbolic interactionist theory has been instrumental in shaping my development as a sociologist. In addition, I thank him for his continued support of my work and for his mischievous sense of humour. I am equally appreciative of the specialist knowledge Professors Pawluch and Cain shared with me. They were, at the time, two of the very few Canadian scholars working in the area of lay participation in alternative health care, and my research would have been the lesser without their counsel. Special thanks to Professor Pawluch, who has been my mentor from the time I began my undergraduate studies in sociology. I am ever grateful to her for her friendship and consistent encouragement.

I would also like to express my appreciation to Althea Prince, Managing Editor of Canadian Scholars' Press, and Rebecca Conolly, Manager of Book Production, both for their commitment to this project and for their thoughtful editorial guidance. Thanks likewise to Rob Baggot, Robert Prus, Mike Saks, Will van den Hoonaard, and the anonymous reviewers of this manuscript, for the constructive suggestions they offered during the proposal stage and editing of this book, as well as to Dirk Lenentine and Denis Desjardins for their essential graphic design skills. In addition, I acknowledge the Social Sciences and Humanities Research Council of Canada and McMaster University for their generous funding of the research on which this book is based.

I am also grateful for the love and support of my family and friends throughout my research and writing. In particular, I thank my father, Doug Low, and my stepmother, Nancy Low, whose confidence in my abilities, and willingness to listen to my on-going analysis, continue to motivate me. I also owe a debt that can never be repaid to Raymond Murphy and Steven Crocker who, along with their friendship, provided me with a place to live and an environment in which I was able to work during a critical point in my life. Last, but never least, my heartfelt thanks to Geoffrey Hudson for his love and his encouragement of my scholarly endeavours—especially this book.

Other friends and colleagues who must be thanked are Jane Abson and Robert McCoy, for their friendship and exemplary research assistance; Justin Busch and Tracey Lee, for reading portions of the manuscript and still remaining my friends; Mary Milliken, for her generous editorial assistance and staunch friendship; Gary Bowden, Sharon Cody, Susan Doherty, Barbara Fisher-Townsend, Deborah Johnston, Lanette Ruff, Vanda Rideout, and Carolyn Williston-Aubie, for their eleventh-hour assistance; Lynn Cameron, for her help in finding participant observation venues and for her enduring friendship; Joey Moore, Catherine Gloor, Scott Anthony Thompson, Rhona Shaw, Elizabeth Graham, Sandy Kitchen, Sally Landon, Jim Mulvale, Heather Young Leslie, Paul Roberts, and Pum van Veldhoven, for their collegiality and camaraderie; Mary Quenville, Rachel Derry, and Rick Miles, for always listening, as well as Nicky Kieffer, for always shining.

Most importantly, I offer my deepest gratitude to the people who participated in this research. In taking part in the interviews they graciously allowed me into their lives. Thus, this book ultimately belongs to them. Finally, my indebtedness to Spirit, which guides me, *Alafia*.

Introduction

Alternative and complementary therapies are a popular form of health care in the Western world (Eisenberg et al. 1993, 1998; Fulder 1996; Health Canada 2001; Lupton 1997). There are numerous therapies available and a variety of commercial outlets stock a plethora of vitamins, herbal remedies, and other types of alternative health care products. A range of venues provides information on healing groups and, in some cases, holistic health associations have centralized access to alternative therapies. Popular media, including television, radio, magazines, and newspapers increasingly feature these approaches to health and healing (Anyinam 1990). For example, in a search of selected popular print media in Canada I found almost four hundred entries for alternative health care between January 1995 and 1997 alone. In addition, there are hundreds of web sites devoted to discussion of alternative and complementary health care on the Internet (Achilles et al. 1999; Coward 1989).

This book concerns the experiences of Canadians who use alternative therapies. The first large-scale survey of the use of alternative approaches among Canadians was carried out by the Canada Health Monitor (1993), who found that 20 percent of Canadians reported participation in alternative forms of healing. Subsequently, in their survey of fifteen thousand Canadians for the Fraser Institute, Ramsay et al. (1999) found that 73 percent of their respondents had used some kind of alternative therapy and de Bruyn (2001) estimated that usership of alternative and complementary therapies amongst Canadians numbers in the millions. Further, it is likely that the use of alternative health care in Canada is under-reported simply because a significant number of people remain reluctant to disclose their use of these therapies to others, especially their doctors (Eisenberg et al. 1998; Low 2000, 2001b; Montbriand and Laing 1991; Ramsay et al. 1999).

The popularity of these therapies amongst Canadians is further evidenced in their self-care spending. For example, a 1997 Angus Reid poll showed that Canadians invested almost $1.8 billion on alternative health care strategies (Angus Reid 1998). De Bruyn (2001:II.23) adds that "in 1996/7, a total of 3.8 billion was spent on complementary and alternative" therapies, including "$1.8 billion on alternative therapies, $937 million on herbs and vitamins, $104 million on special diet programs, and more than $998 million on books, classes, and equipment." The Fraser Institute (Achilles et al. 1999) reports that in 1999 the most frequently used alternative therapies in Canada were chiropractic (36 percent), relaxation techniques (23 percent), massage (23 percent), prayer (21 percent), herbal therapies (17 percent), special diets (12 percent), folk remedies (12 percent), acupuncture (12 percent), yoga (10 percent), and homeopathy (8 percent).

Additional evidence for the popularity of alternative health care in Canada includes the number of courses in alternative therapies available. For instance, in September of 1998 one Canadian community college held weekend workshops and courses on a variety of therapies, including ear candling, mystical healing gems, herbalism, homeopathy, Chinese medicine, and *shiatsu* massage (Mohawk College 1998:156–59). By 2003, the same college not only offered several workshops or courses in complementary therapies, but also provided a certificate programme in aromatherapy, and was in the process of developing a diploma programme in herbal medicine (Mohawk College 2003a, 2003b).

There is also evidence that participation in alternative therapies in Canada is on the rise (Achilles et al. 1999; de Bruyn 2001). For example, Northcott and Bachynsky (1993:432) found that "annual usage of alternative health care therapies (other than chiropractic) ... increased from 1979 to 1988;" and de Bruyn (2001:II.21) reports "notable increases" in the use of chiropractic, massage, herbalism, acupuncture, homeopathy, and reflexology between 1993 and 1996. Likewise, the number of alternative and complementary therapists in Canada has increased, and it is estimated that there are approximately twelve thousand licensed alternative practitioners in Canada (Achilles et al. 1999). The number of actual alternative and complementary practitioners in Canada is impossible to determine, as many practitioners—such as aromatherapists or *reiki* practitioners—remain unregulated and undocumented. Clearly, alternative therapies are an important part of Canadians' health care regimes and their use of these approaches to health care is deserving of deeper analysis.

Despite the number of people participating in alternative approaches to health and health care, very few sociologists have examined individuals' experiences in using these therapies. It is with this issue that I am concerned in this book. Rather than focussing on alternative practitioners or the therapies themselves, this book provides the reader with a detailed understanding of the subjective experiences of the Canadian user of alternative approaches to health and healing. I explore how and why the people who took part in this research come to use alternative therapies, the ideology that informs the alternative models of health and healing they espouse, and the impact on them of the ideology underpinning these models.

The people who spoke with me sought out alternative health care in order to solve problems for which they found little or no redress in other quarters. They began using alternative therapies through a variety of different points of *entrée*, including encounters with friends, family members, and the media, among others. Once involved in using these therapies, they developed ever-expanding networks of alternative health care composed of alternative practitioners and lay users of alternative therapies. In participating in alternative health care, and in interaction with others who use it, these people began to take on alternative ideologies of health and healing. For some, these ideologies became a mechanism through which they transformed their subjective perceptions of health status for the better. Quite simply, despite experiencing what is serious physical disability or disease, these people are able to see themselves as healthy because they are engaged in the process of healing. Others became so enamoured of alternative ideology that they sought training to become alternative practitioners themselves.

However, there are other, less beneficial, consequences to self and identity inherent in adopting these models of health and healing. For instance, while participation in these therapies allows these people a measure of control over their health care, adoption of alternative health and healing ideology means that they must assume total responsibility for any problems of ill health they experience. Moreover, persistent social inequality means that the benefits to self these people experience are not available to those Canadians without the financial and other resources necessary to participate in alternative approaches to health care. Furthermore, in all cases, these people had to manage the deviant identities they acquired through their use of alternative therapies.

THE STUDY

A symbolic interactionist understanding of the individual and society informs the analysis I present in this book. This perspective is particularly appropriate to the questions I address, as my intent is a subjectivist understanding of the experiences of lay people who use alternative health care. Symbolic interactionism was useful in this research, since what distinguishes it from structuralist approaches is its focus on the micro level of society, its concern with the subjective experiences of individuals in interaction, and its emphasis on individuals' own understandings of reality as a basis for their actions (Blumer 1969). In giving meaning to symbols, the individual is able to interpret the actions of others, conceive his or her own course of action, and anticipate future actions. As individuals interact with each other, meanings become shared, thus allowing people to communicate with each other through the use of significant symbols, such as language, gestures, and appearance. Meaning is not inherent in symbols; rather, it is a negotiated and social product, therefore symbols can hold a multiplicity of meanings. Symbolic interactionism's subjectivist orientation permits the researcher to gain insight into the processes by which individuals both create, and modify, meaning (Blumer 1969; Maines 1981).

Moreover, a qualitative research design was the natural choice for this research, as it ensures that the focus remains on the individual, emphasizing "the value of the person's own story" (Becker 1996:vi). Such a focus allowed me to form an interpretive understanding of the motives and meanings behind individuals' participation in alternative approaches to health and healing (Becker 1966). Specifically, I used unstructured interviews as a primary means of data gathering (McCraken 1988).[1] I also collected data through participant observation and review of a variety of printed materials. In total, twenty-one people participated in this research. Sufficient interviews were conducted such that themes and patterns in the data were confirmed by informant after informant (Glaser and Strauss 1967).[2] I recruited informants using purposeful sampling, employing snowball and convenience techniques (Babbie 1986).[3] In addition to approaching individuals independently, I placed flyers describing the study in the Wellness Centre,[4] a local holistic health care facility frequented by some of the people who took part in this research; a naturopath's office; and a local natural food store. As part of my field notes, I kept track of how I made contact with each informant, enabling me to note any patterns in the data which were a result of friendship or other networks (see Figure 0.1).

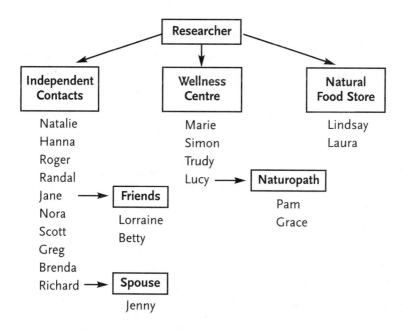

Figure 0.1. Informant Contact Network

The interviews ranged anywhere from an hour to an hour and a half in length. I also conducted follow-up interviews whenever necessary. All the interviews were tape recorded and fully transcribed.[5] Informants were asked to choose the location of the interview and the majority of them opted to speak with me in their homes. Informant preference to be interviewed in the home proved advantageous: in addition to allowing them to be more candid than in other locations, in the privacy of their homes many informants felt comfortable demonstrating various therapeutic techniques involved in the alternative health care they use. I began each interview by asking informants variations of the general question: How did you first become involved in using alternative therapies? I then concentrated on listening, probing to explore issues informants raised and to seek clarification, and noting when there were pauses in the conversation. As Becker (1970b:193) points out, statements volunteered by informants are "likely to reflect the observer's preoccupations and possible biases less than [those] made in response to" questions posed by the researcher. Thus, the use of unstructured interviews enhanced the validity of this analysis.

Validity in this research also rests on the *richness* of the data collected. The sheer amount of information provided by informants guards against researcher bias "by making it difficult for the observer to restrict ... observations so that he [or she] sees only what supports his [or her] prejudices and expectations" (Becker 1970a:52). The validity of this research was also confirmed by informant review of the findings ensuring that my analysis reflects their beliefs about, and experiences of participation in, alternative approaches to health and healing.

Also, when theory is "induced from diverse data," the researcher is less likely to impose his/her perceptions of reality on the phenomena at hand (Glaser and Strauss 1967:239). Thus the rigour of this study was enhanced through the use of a variety of sources of information in addition to the primary interview data. This information complements the interview data in a variety of ways (Shaffir and Stebbins 1991). For example, my own experiences as a user of alternative therapies provides me with insider awareness that reinforces the validity of this research (Douglas 1976). Further, the participant observation I conducted gave me a deeper familiarity with the various alternative therapies these informants used and practised, including acupuncture, aromatherapy, astrological healing, *bagua*, Chinese herbal medicine, chiropractic, Christian Science medicine, creative visualization, crystal healing, ear candling, Feldenkrais method, herbal medicine, homeopathy, hypnotherapy, massage, meditation, midwifery, naturopathy, psychic healing, reflexology, *reiki*, the results system, therapeutic touch, vitamin therapy, and yoga—as well as fasting and a variety of other dietary regimes.

In the same way, participant observation made me aware of the alternative health care remedies and products that were locally available to informants. For instance, in the spring of 1995 I participated in a yoga session specially designed for people with multiple sclerosis. Later that year I attended an open house at the Wellness Centre, a holistic health centre providing several types of alternative therapies, including *reiki*, acupuncture, ear candling, reflexology, and aromatherapy, as well as *shiatsu* and Swedish massage. During this open-house I was able to speak with several of the alternative healers who practised out of the centre and to experience several therapies myself. During March of 1997 I attended a local healing fair that had exhibits on vitamins and minerals, ear candling, homeopathy, reflexology, *reiki*, crystal healing, and aromatherapy massage, among other products and therapeutic techniques. I also spent time exploring commercial venues that stocked many of the alternative healing books, products, and remedies used by people who participated in this research. In addition, I reviewed advertising material, popular books, and pamphlets describing the various alternative therapies used by informants, as well as a number of magazines devoted to alternative approaches to health and healing.

In contrast to the goal of most quantitative measures, which is to "continually yield an unvarying measurement" (Kirk and Miller 1986:41–42), the test of the reliability of qualitative methods is that they generate "similar observations within the same time period." In other words, although studying the same setting, different researchers will naturally observe different things at different times (Becker 1970a). It is important to note that it is that things have changed over time, not that the measure is unreliable. Furthermore, even observations that are collected within the same time period are "rarely identical ... but rather ... are consistent with respect to the particular features of interest to the observer" (Kirk and Miller 1986:42). For example, the words used by these informants often varied; however, they remained thematically and theoretically consistent. For instance, although one informant might have talked about the inner self, and another about the higher self, they were both describing how they tap into their spiritual power to heal themselves. The reliability of this study was also enhanced through the constant comparison of a series of interviews, where each interview served to validate or refine the conclusions drawn from data collected in the others (Trow 1970); as well as through the use of field notes and analytic notes which allowed me to track the emergence of themes and patterns in the data.

I take a grounded theory approach in this research, meaning that rather than beginning with theoretical assumptions and then seeking data that conform to them, theory emerges through the process of empirical research (Corbin and Strauss 1990; Glaser and Strauss 1967). In addition, grounded theory analysis assumes that data analysis is ongoing through-out the research process, from recruitment and data collection through to theoretical sampling of the literature and final writing-up of the findings (Strauss and Corbin 1990). I analysed the data for this research using the technique of open coding, which is "the process of breaking down, examining, comparing, conceptualizing, and categorizing data" (Strauss and Corbin 1990:61). By making comparisons within and asking questions about the data, emergent patterns are noted that in turn contribute to theory-building (Glaser and Strauss 1967; Strauss and Corbin 1990). For example, the alternative model of health these informants espouse rests on the notion of holism, which for them is the unity of body, mind, and spirit. Thus, holism emerged as an overarching theme in the analysis (see Figure 0.2).

Through the process of comparative coding, the categories of balance and control emerged within the theme of holism and were broken down into several concepts and sub-concepts. For instance, the analytic category of balance contains two concepts: balance in the body and balance in the self. These concepts were further broken down into several sub-concepts based on convergences and divergences between informants' beliefs about how unity of mind, body, and spirit is achieved through balance. Thus the concept of balance in the body expanded to include the sub-concepts of balancing physiological systems and balancing bodily energy, both of which are related to the sub-concept of listening to the body. Balance in the self includes the sub-concept of being grounded or centred. The concepts of balance in the body and balance in the self are inextricably connected to the category of control, which is itself composed of two distinct concepts: taking control and self-control, where taking control includes the sub-concepts of

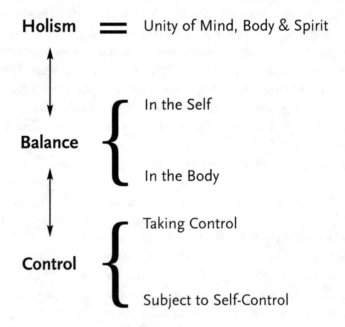

Figure 0.2. An Alternative Model of Health

control of one's healing process and taking responsibility for one's health. Finally, the concept of self-control is comprised of such sub-concepts as control over one's behaviour and lifestyle choices, and control over one's thought processes and emotional reactions.

THE STRUCTURE OF THE BOOK

In chapter one I begin the story of the experiences of these informants by addressing the questions of how we should conceptualize alternative health care and just who we should consider a user of alternative therapies. In it I argue for a subjectivist understanding of alternative approaches to health and healing, as well as against the notion that the individual who participates in alternative forms of healing is a particular *type* of person. Using demographic information collected from the people who took part in this study and comparing it with what is known in general about the users of alternative therapies in Canada, the United States (US), and the United Kingdom (UK), I demonstrate that people who use these therapies are no different from individuals engaged in any other form of health-seeking behaviour.

In the next two chapters I consider how and why people participate in alternative approaches to health and healing. Through analysis of the networks of alternative therapy use negotiated by these informants, I present a new conceptual model of the health care system informed by their experiences. Rather than conceptualizing alternative therapies as isolated, this model situates alternative forms of healing within every sector of the health care system. In chapter three I examine the debates surrounding what is said to motivate the individual to seek out alternative modes of health and healing. I demonstrate how it is more fruitful to understand individuals' use of alternative therapies as a generic social process of problem-solving than it is to focus on particular ideological motivating factors.

Chapters four and five are the lynchpins of this book, as they contain the alternative models of health and healing espoused by the people who participated in this research. The centrality of these models to understanding the experiences of individuals who participate in alternative therapies lies in the link they provide between adoption of alternative health belief systems and the impact of these alternative health and healing ideologies on an individual's sense of self. In chapter four I describe these informants' model of alternative healing and discuss how they give meaning to it by contrasting it with what they see as the negative standard of biomedicine. In chapter five I turn to an analysis of their model of alternative health. This model gives voice to the lay perspective, in contrast to existing models of alternative health which rely on physician and alternative practitioner beliefs.[6] I continue with a critical analysis of the meaning these informants give to the conceptual categories of holism, balance, and control which make up their alternative model of health, and conclude with an examination of the implications for the individual of adopting such an approach to health and healing.

I extend my analysis of the potential implications for the individual of participation in alternative health care in chapter six by addressing the hitherto underdeveloped analysis of the relationship between alternative therapy use and the self. I discuss how some of the people who spoke with me used the ideology contained within this model of health to construct a healthy sense of self. In chapter seven I address the less positive impact of alternative healing ideology on identity through analysis of how these people manage the stigma associated with their participation in alternative therapies.

My conclusion provides a summary of the major findings of this research, a discussion of the implications of these findings for health policy, and suggestions for future research in the growing field of the sociology of alternative forms of health and healing. I have also included an appendix of brief descriptions of the alternative therapies mentioned in this book. It is important to note that I provide these sketches solely for the benefit of those readers who may be unfamiliar with particular alternative healing techniques; in no way do I mean these descriptions to be read as definitive. Hence I have chosen the descriptions randomly from a selection of scholarly literature, popular sources, advertising pamphlets, and—in keeping with my focus on the user of alternative therapies—quotations from informant interviews.

NOTES

1. The interviews took place between 1993 and 1996 and the transcription was conducted between 1993 and 1998.
2. The number of informants who participate in grounded theory research is in one sense irrelevant, as the unit of analysis in these cases is the concept rather than the individual (Corbin and Strauss 1990).

3. All informants were asked to give their written consent prior to the interviews. They were informed of the purpose of the research, assured that their participation in the study was voluntary, told that they had the right to end the interview at any time and that they were not required to answer any questions they did not wish to. They were also made aware that if they decided to withdraw from the project at any time, their tapes and transcripts would be destroyed. Participants were offered an opportunity to review their transcripts and those sections of the analysis containing portions of their interviews. Informants' identities remain protected through the use of pseudonyms, which has the advantage of presenting them as people rather than data.
4. The Wellness Centre is a pseudonym.
5. Quotations from the interview transcripts appearing in this book are given verbatim and have only been edited for clarity of meaning, or in one instance at the request of an informant whose words have been edited for idiomatic consistency. This person spoke in pronounced Cockney idiom and felt misrepresented as uneducated in the transcript of her interview.
6. See Cain et al. (1999) and Lowenberg (1992) for alternative and complementary healing ideology from the practitioner perspective.

CHAPTER ONE

What Are Alternative Therapies and Who Uses Them?[1]

Two conceptual problems I encountered early on in this research were to determine just what to class as an alternative therapy and just who to consider a user of alternative health care. That conceptualizing alternative therapy is problematic is evident from a cursory review of the relevant literature, which reveals a "maze of definitions" where alternative approaches to health and healing are concerned (Achilles 2001:I.8; Eskinazi 1998). In short, there is no consensus as to how we should refer to these forms of health care. Given this definitional conundrum, determining who is a user of alternative therapies also proves problematic.

WHAT ARE ALTERNATIVE THERAPIES?

Anyinam (1990:69) pointedly illustrates the ambiguity inherent in conceptualizations of alternative health care when he writes: "'Alternative medicine' ... has been variously termed 'complementary medicine,' 'traditional medicine,' 'holistic medicine,' 'unorthodox medicine,' 'fringe/marginal medicine,' 'folk medicine,' and 'ethnomedicine.'" In addition to these concepts, Health Canada (2001) and Casey and Picherack (2001) have abbreviated alternative and complementary health care as CAHC. The acronym CAM (complementary and alternative medicine) is also increasingly used to refer to these approaches to health and healing (Blais 2000; Kelner et al. 2000; White and Ernst 2001).

What all of these concepts have in common is that they define alternative therapies in terms of what they are not, namely, allopathic medicine (Furnham and Bhagrath 1993).[2] For example, McGuire (1988:3) defines alternative healing as "a wide range of beliefs and practices that adherents expect to affect health but that are not promulgated by medical personnel in the dominant biomedical system." Ten years later, Eisenberg et al. (1998:1569) reiterate that these therapies may be "functionally defined as interventions neither taught widely in medical schools nor generally available in US hospitals." Similarly, Kelner and Wellman (2000) define CAM relative to medical practice. They write that CAM is "an approach to health care that while different from conventional medicine, is sometimes complementary to it and at other times distinctly alternative" (Kelner and Wellman 2000:5–6).

In addition, from the perspective of medical professionals, alternative therapy refers to those approaches that fall outside of medical practice (Kelner and Wellman 2000). More specifically, that a particular therapy has not been legitimated by the medical community. For example, Knipchild et al. (1990:626) analysed general practitioners' beliefs about the effectiveness of alternative therapies and found that "many Dutch GPs believe in the efficacy of common alternative procedures" including acupuncture, manual therapy, and homeopathy. However, some alternative therapies, such as iridology and astrological healing, were not seen as credible in the eyes of the general practitioners they studied. They write: "Manual therapy in the Netherlands is generally not considered alternative medicine any more. No less than 80% believes [sic] it to be efficacious in the treatment of patients with chronic neck or back problems" (Knipchild et al. 1990:625). A similar distinction is made by Leech (1999), a principal medical officer of Britain's National Health Service Executive, who equates complementary therapies with those that have become regulated and whose efficacy has been certified according to medical and scientific standards. Researchers who favour such functionalist or residual definitions tend to categorize particular therapies "along a spectrum that varies from 'more alternative' to 'less alternative' in relationship to existing medical school curricula, clinical training, and practice" (Eisenberg et al. 1998:1574; Northcott 1994).

However, as Sharma (1992:4) notes: "'medical' practices can never be sharply distinguished from 'non-medical' practices in reality." For instance, alternative practitioners often adopt and incorporate various biomedical concepts within their health and healing paradigm (Northcott 1994; Sharma 1993). As Simon, a former medical student who practices acupuncture, told me, "I can understand the release of endorphins and all the chemicals from the brain. The analgesic effect of acupuncture, the calming effect; different chemicals are released." Further, incorporation of biomedical concepts within the education of alternative practitioners has long been a strategy used by them in their efforts to professionalize (Boon 1998); and the medical community continues to adopt concepts and therapies used by alternative practitioners (Achilles 2001; Northcott 1994; Saks 1997b; Sharma 1992, 1993; Tataryn and Verhoef 2001). For example, there is increasing talk of a holistic or integrative approach to allopathic medicine; many alternative therapies are part of medical school curriculum; and a variety of alternative therapies are available in hospitals (de Bruyn 2001; O'Connor 1995; Sharma 1992; Tataryn and Verhoef 2001).

Given the overlap between alternative and allopathic concepts and therapeutic techniques, defining alternative health and healing residually is hardly useful (Wardwell 1994). To further muddy the conceptual waters, what is considered an alternative therapy changes over time (Bakx 1991; Wardwell 1994), from social context to social context, and from person to person (Boon et al. 1999; Low 2001a). For instance, several of the people who participated in this research referred to the variable definitional boundaries surrounding alternative therapies. In Roger's words:

> One of the things I got involved in a very long time ago is considered part of the alternative medicine alphabet soup of things, but at that time I didn't think of it that way. A lot of these things, where the boundary is, what gets included under that rubric, is kind of fluid.

Clearly, objectivist definitions of alternative therapies are inherently problematic (Low 2001a; Pawluch 1996; Sharma 1993; Thomas et al. 2001). Equally troubling is Jones' (1987) conclusion that there is no real difference between alternative and allopathic medicine. Citing the British Medical Association's Report on Alternative Medicine, Jones (1987:69) argues that "there ... is no logical class of 'alternative therapies': there are only therapies with or without good evidence for their efficacy." He writes that "time, touch, and compassion ... are features of all good medical practice, and exclusive to none" (Jones 1987:69). However, the people who participated in this research do believe that there is something distinctive about their alternative health care.

How then can we write meaningfully about alternative therapies? Pawluch (1996) argues that defining alternative health and healing objectively is impossible. She concludes that the only viable definitional strategy is to look at the claims that people make about what is and what isn't alternative health care. One group of claims are those made by alternative practitioners (Lowenberg 1992). Other claims are made by medical professionals (Eisenberg et al. 1993) and academics (Aakster 1986). Claims that often receive less attention are those made by lay people. It is these latter claims that are the focus of my analysis.

The people who took part in this research referred to their participation in alternative forms of health care in a variety of ways, including alternative therapy/medicine, complementary therapy/medicine, holistic health care, and natural healing. However, I have chosen to use variations of "alternative therapy," over CAM or complementary therapy/medicine, for several reasons. First of all, as is the case with the concept of alternative therapy, there is no consistent meaning given to the terms "complementary therapy" or "complementary medicine." For instance, Fulder and Munro (1985:545) cite a definition where complementary means that both alternative and allopathic therapeutic approaches have "separate areas of competence" and that complementary therapies are neither "alternative [nor] supplementary to conventional medicine" (Fulder and Munro 1985:542). Other researchers define complementary therapy as the concurrent use of both alternative and allopathic forms of health care (Cant and Sharma 1995; Northcott and Bachynsky 1993; Sharma 1992) or therapies that are subsidiary and additional to medicine (Murray and Shepherd 1993). From the perspective of alternative practitioners, complementary can mean additional, subsidiary, supplementary, or alternative to medicine (Cant and Calnan 1991). Examples taken from research focussing on the users of alternative therapies provide still other definitions. For example, Pawluch et al. (1994) found that the people who participated in their research used alternative therapies as part of an overall self-care strategy which they referred to as a complementary approach to health care. For these informants, the word "complementary" has a precise meaning. It means that they do not choose between systems of health care; rather, they use whichever therapeutic modalities they feel can help them without assigning superiority to one system over the other.

Secondly, while all of the people I spoke with use both alternative and allopathic therapies, often for the same problem, they do not do so in a precisely complementary manner, if to complement means that one thing enhances another. Nor was their use of these therapies resonant with a definition of "complementary" meant to suggest that such an approach to healing is simply a matter of putting together health care teams out of the myriad options available. Nor is it one that assumes that co-operative relations between alternative and allopathic practitioners are easy to achieve, as implied by a definition employing a notion of compatibility. Indeed, almost all informants told me of their struggles in trying to find a medical doctor who would work co-operatively with their alternative practitioners. Greg's and Grace's experiences typify the frustrations expressed by most other informants. For example, Grace told me: "My naturopath would be more than happy to speak to my GP. My GP just doesn't think that he has any reason to talk to her." And Greg said:

> That's where I tried to get them to interact.... My [chiropractor] was the one that first discovered the pinched nerve and I guess it took months for him to even get the GP's attention, leaving messages with him, just trying to get him to talk to him about it.

In the end, most of the participants in this study settled for a physician who would tolerate, if not support, their use of alternative therapies. For instance, Jane said: "[My doctor] doesn't want to know about the chiropractor. If I go to [one], that's my business. He doesn't want to hear about it."

In addition, many of the people who spoke with me understand their dual use of alternative and allopathic health care in a purely instrumental way, such as in cases where they need access to medical technology for which health care professionals remain the sole gatekeepers (Conrad and Schneider 1980). For example, Lucy needed the services of a medical doctor for certain diagnostic tests. In her words, "I went to the naturopath and had her recommend a medical doctor and so now when lab tests have to be taken [it] is out of one realm into the other one." Similarly, Jenny said: "I actually should get [a GP] because the dentist requires it. I did have one because I had to have my rabies injections. I just went to see him to get some jabs." And finally, Hanna told me she seeks out medical care "only for blood work and annual check-ups." In short, the stories informants told about their dual use of alternative and allopathic therapies did not sound particularly complementary according to any conventional meanings attributed to the term, and are more rightly conceptualized as accounts of concurrent use of allopathic and alternative approaches to health care.

A third reason, and one more important to the arguments I make here, is that only two informants, who were not also practitioners, used the word complementary, whether in describing their use of alternative therapies and/or their concurrent use of alternative and allopathic health care. More precisely, of the twenty-one people I interviewed, only seven used the term complementary at all. Of those seven, five were, or were in training to become, alternative practitioners. To illustrate, the two lay informants who used the concept of complementary did not define it in the same way. Richard's use of the concept focuses on compatibility, whereas Laura's definition of complementary rests on the notion of enhancement. According to Richard, "It isn't that one's better than the other. They are, in fact, compatible. And they're complementary to each, one and other." In contrast, Laura phrased it this way: "When somebody's sick and they're going through chemotherapy, any type of cancer therapy, or any type of hard-on-the-body treatment, I would say complement with vitamins or that type of things." While two examples are not enough to draw definitive conclusions, when coupled with the lack of use of the concept of complementary by all other lay users who participated in this study, they are enough to seriously question the wholesale use of the concept in describing individuals' use of alternative and/or dual use of allopathic and alternative therapies.

Furthermore, those informants who identified as alternative practitioners did not use the concept of complementary as a synonym for alternative therapy, as is seen in a great deal of the relevant literature (Furnham and Beard 1995; Furnham and Bhagrath 1993; Furnham and Kirkcaldy 1996; Furnham et al. 1995; Vincent and Furnham 1996). Rather, Scott told me that there are three different forms of therapy at issue: alternative, allopathic, and complementary—a distinction researchers sometimes obliquely allude to, though rarely, if ever, explain (Furnham and Forey 1994). What is significant about the following excerpt from Scott's interview is that he equates complementary therapy with alternative therapies which have become almost indistinguishable from allopathic practice.

> There's two broad categories. The first one is mainstream or allopathic medicine.... Then [you've] got the other category which is alternative and within this I would make a division between [two types of alternative therapy]. There's a part of alternative medicine that can be seen as a complement to traditional allopathic medicine.... You have some people from the more conservative part of the alternative health field who would fall into this category. Maybe a naturopath, a chiropractor. You know chiropractors are some of the most allopathically oriented practitioners that you could possibly have.... You can be so mainstream if you're a chiropractor. Basically you could be a mechanic for the body or else you could be out there in the land of healing.

It is ironic that Scott's definition of complementary is commensurate, albeit for very different reasons, with one frequently made by members of the allopathic medical community: namely, that complementary therapies are alternative therapies that have been legitimated by medical science (Knipchild et al. 1990; Leech 1999).

Haviland (1992) asserts that rather than reflecting a genuine partnering of alternative and allopathic approaches, the concept of complementarity has increasingly come into use for largely political reasons. Similarly, Cant and Calnan (1991:44) conclude that the claim that "practitioners are offering an alternative and the idea that the role is one of 'complement' to orthodoxy may be overstated." Of the practitioners they interviewed, only one naturopath saw himself in what they term a truly complementary role. While some of the practitioners they spoke with described their role as only supplementary to allopathic medicine, most who used "a notion of complementary" did so in ways which belied pragmatic concerns rather than co-operative teamwork (Cant and Calnan 1991:46). For example, these practitioners used the concept in describing their dependence on general practitioners for client referral. Likewise, I argue that the use of the concept of complementary, amongst the alternative practitioners who participated in this research, is reflective of their experiences interacting with medical professionals who continue to dominate the healing professions (Saks 1998). Specifically, these alternative practitioners have a professional interest in using the concept both to avoid the appearance of competition with physicians and to reduce the likelihood that they will be labelled "quacks." For instance, Hanna, a yoga practitioner, frames her approach in complementary terms, stating that alternative practitioners and allopathic physicians have different areas of expertise:

> I like to think of it as complementary medicine, but we complement them [doctors]. There are certain medical things that I just can not do and things that they can not do, so I think we complement one another and I think we should be accepted on that aspect rather than as quacks.

Similarly, throughout her interview, Marie, a *reiki* practitioner, took pains to present herself as a collaborator rather than a competitor with allopathic medicine. However, it is clear that she sees allopathic medicine as subsidiary to alternative therapy. One is not enhancing the other; rather, allopathic medicine is used solely in an auxiliary capacity. She said: "Not disregarding mainstream medicine. They can work hand in hand. We like to call them complementary therapies. If for some reason the natural remedies are not working, by all means see a physician."

Having just made the case that the concept of complementary therapy is not one that necessarily emerges out of lay perspectives on health and healing, I must address the fact that some researchers have noted that their informants do use the concept of complementary. As noted above, Pawluch et al. (1994) found that their informants used it to describe an approach to health care where they make use of a variety of therapies and where they do not make evaluative distinctions between allopathic and alternative approaches to healing. On one level my findings are in stark contrast to those of Pawluch et al. (1994). Not only were almost all of the lay informants I spoke with inclined to make evaluative statements about different forms of health care—including assigning superiority to alternative over allopathic approaches—as previously noted, but also only two used the concept of complementary therapy at any time throughout their interviews. However, on another level, their findings support my arguments here, as Pawluch et al. (1994) use the concept of complementary in their research precisely because their informants do. Similarly, I have purposefully chosen to use in my analysis variations of "alternative therapy," rather than CAM or complementary therapies, because these variations more accurately reflect the beliefs and experiences of the lay people who shared their stories of participation in alternative approaches to health and healing with me.

WHO USES ALTERNATIVE THERAPIES?

The ambiguous nature of the concept of alternative therapy was brought home to me repeatedly when making initial contact with potential research participants. Almost everyone who telephoned me referred to the blurry boundaries surrounding what is and what isn't an alternative health care. Most often this uncertainty took the form of an exchange whereby they began by telling me how interested they were in taking part in the interviews, but almost immediately said things such as, "I'm not really sure if I belong in your study" (Pam). I continued these conversations by asking potential research recruits if they considered themselves users of alternative therapies. They almost always responded by asking me to tell them if they were. For instance, Scott said, "I guess it sort of depends on what *you* define as alternative therapies" (his emphasis). Invariably, my response was that if they thought it was, it was.

Furthermore, any attempt to classify people as users of alternative therapies on the basis of non-use of allopathic medicine is problematic, since rarely, if ever, do people participate in alternative therapies to the exclusion of biomedicine,[3] and all the people who took part in this research made use of both alternative and allopathic health care. Another aspect of this problem is whether or not people are exclusively lay users or also practitioners of alternative therapies. One must point out that it is not uncommon for people to begin by participating in alternative health care in order to address their own health problems and then later seek training to practice alternative therapies on others (Sharma 1992), as did several of the people who participated in this research. However, all these people began by using the therapies for themselves and continue to employ them as part of their personal health care regimes. This type of overlap between user and practitioner roles can be partially explained through one aspect of alternative health and healing ideology, namely, the notion of self-healing (Furnham 1994; Lowenberg 1992). According to Natalie, an informant who both uses and practices alternative therapies: "It's up to the individual who wants to heal themselves…. Everybody can heal themselves if they want to." While I am not trying to make the case that all users of alternative therapies necessarily become practitioners, I am suggesting that it makes no sense to necessarily exclude people from analysis of lay use of alternative health care because they may also identify themselves as practitioners or healers. The only way to resolve these epistemological problems, while remaining consistent with a subjectivist perspective, is to consider people users of alternative therapies if they so identify.

Is There An Alternative Therapy Type?

Fifteen women and six men took part in this study. In general this distribution reflects the higher female rates of participation in alternative health care reported in Canada (Achilles et al. 1999), the US (Eisenberg et al. 1998) and the UK (Fulder 1996). As Sharma (1990:128) concludes: "There is consistent evidence that higher proportions of alternative medicine patients are female."[4] For instance, 21 percent of Canadian women, in contrast to 17 percent of Canadian men, used alternative health care in 2000/2001 (Canadian Institute for Health Information 2002; Gill 2003) and according to the Canada Health Monitor (1993), among a sub-sample[5] of users of alternative health therapies they surveyed, the female/male ratio was one point five to one. Similarly, in their UK study, Thomas et al. (2001) found that just over 56 percent of female and 43 percent of males reported using alternative therapies. The male/female gap in user-ship is narrower in the US with 52 percent of women and 48 percent of men reporting participation in alternative health care (Eisenberg et al. 1998).

However, Eisenberg et al. (1993:248, 1998) argue that there are "no significant differences according to sex" in their US research and Northcott and Bachynsky (1993) found that the female/male ratio in their Canadian study was almost one to one. Further, Blais (2000) reports that male participation in alternative therapies is on the rise in Quebec. It is also likely that male rates of usership of alternative health care are under-represented in much of the research on these therapies. Males are vulnerable to under-representation if only for the fact that many men are unwilling to discuss issues relating to their health and health care, and are therefore less likely to take part in research concerned with such issues (Trypuc 1994).[6] In addition, it is well documented that women access all forms of health care more frequently than men do (Miller and Findlay 1994). Thus whether one is male or female has less to do with participation in alternative therapies than it does with gendered patterns of health-seeking behaviour in general.

The people who spoke with me ranged in age from twenty-six to fifty-nine years, with fourteen of them falling between forty-one and fifty-nine years of age. This age distribution is similar to findings reported in the literature on alternative therapy use in the West up until the mid-1990s. In Canada, research shows that usership of alternative health care is distributed over the lifespan; however, the majority of those participating in alternative therapies are aged between thirty and forty-five years (Blais 2000; Wellman 1995). Similarly, in the US, Glik (1988) concludes that participation in alternative therapies is most frequent among the middle-aged. For example, Eisenberg et al. (1993:248) found that "the use of unconventional therapy in the US is significantly more common among people twenty-five to forty-nine years of age" than in any other age groups. In a later study, Eisenberg et al. (1998) report that most users of alternative therapies fall in the thirty-five to fifty year range. And in their UK study of people using acupuncture, homeopathy, or osteopathy, Vincent and Furnham's (1996:40) subjects ranged in age from thirty-eight to forty-seven years.

While the ages of the people who spoke with me correspond to the findings in this literature, I have my suspicions that they under-represent participation in alternative health care among young people. For instance, more recent national surveys in Canada indicate that the highest rate of usership is among those in younger age groups (Achilles et al. 1999). More specifically, Ramsay et al. (1999) report that the most frequent participation in alternative therapies is amongst those eighteen to twenty-four years old. In addition, studies of users of these therapies tend to focus on the clients of chiropractors, naturopaths, and homeopathists. However, due to their youth, users of alternative therapies under thirty have fewer occasions to visit practitioners who specialize in muscular/skeletal problems such as chiropractors. Moreover, young people may be unable to afford the fees charged by alternative practitioners such as naturopaths or homeopaths. Yet people under thirty years of age may well identify themselves as users of alternative therapies when they buy Echinacea, or practice yoga, or participate in meditation as forms of self-care. Thus age is more likely an indicator of consumption of health care in general, and of the ability to pay for alternative therapy, than it is reflective of whether or not someone uses alternative therapies.

All of the informants in this study were white. Eighteen identified themselves as Canadians of British or Celtic heritage; two were British; and one, while born in Poland, grew up in Holland and Kenya. Likewise, national survey research from the US reports that up to 82 percent of those who use alternative therapies are white (Eisenberg et al. 1998). However, this is not to imply that using alternative approaches to health and health care is restricted to whites. For example, the informants who took part in Pawluch et al.'s (1998b) study of people coping with HIV/AIDS through the use of complementary therapy came from a diverse range of ethnic and racial backgrounds. Furthermore, the relationship between use of alternative approaches to health and healing and ethnic background is greatly dependent on cultural context (Low 2001b). For instance, Asians who make use of Chinese herbal medicine may well define it as traditional rather than alternative and would thus be under-represented in surveys of alternative health care use.

All but two of the participants in this research identified themselves as middle class or upper-middle class, and all had completed some form of post-secondary education. These demographic characteristics are consistent with the bulk of Canadian research (Blais 2000; Canada Health Monitor 1993; Northcott and Bachynsky 1993; Ramsay et al. 1999). A similar pattern is found in the US (O'Connor 1995). For instance, Eisenberg et al.(1993:248, 1998) found that use of alternative therapies is "significantly more common among persons with a college education," and

McGuire and Kantor (1987:221) conclude "that nonmedical forms of healing are ... rather widespread among educated, fully acculturated, economically secure people." In the UK people who participate in alternative therapies come predominately from the professional classes (Fulder 1996).

However, Sharma (1990:128) argues that studies have found only slight variations in socio-economic status (SES) between users of alternative therapies and the general population, and in some cases "no differences at all." Furthermore, many surveys concerned with the use of alternative therapies contain questions about visits to alternative practitioners, the most expensive participation in these approaches to health care (Fulder and Munro 1985). Therefore, the finding that those in higher SES ranges use alternative health care more frequently is more likely a reflection of their ability to pay rather than a lack of desire for alternative approaches to health and healing on the part of those in lower SES categories.

The informants in this study came from a variety of religious backgrounds. Six identified themselves as Protestant and six as agnostic or as having no religion. Three are Buddhist, two practice Wicca, two are Catholic, and one is Mennonite. This distribution of religious affiliation is similar to that found by Wellman (1995) in her Canadian study of clients of chiropractors and therapists who practice the Alexander technique. It is also consistent with the Canada Health Monitor's (1993:124) findings that most respondents who answered yes to the question, "In the past six months, have you used any of the following alternative therapies?" reported that they had no religion or espouse a religion outside mainstream Judaeo-Christian faiths. Moreover, while fifteen of the people who spoke with me identified themselves as belonging to one or other form of Christianity, or as having no religion, it became clear during the interviews that nine of these people also espoused what Creedon (1998:44) calls "pastiche spirituality or religion à la carte," what I call, for lack of a better term, new age spirituality. For example, Lorraine described her religious beliefs as follows:

> The whole point of being born on earth is to grow in your spirituality. Each person is on that particular rung of the ladder; when you're ready to learn, your teacher will enter your life. I am Anglican, but whoever went to church on the street, that's who I went with. So I've been to Salvation Army, Delta Tabernacle, United, Methodist, Catholic. But this has helped me. I have not become mind-locked into any religion. God is here in my heart. God is within me, not in some building.

Similarly, Marie told me that while she was brought up a Catholic, she now follows her own spiritual path. In her words: "I'm a recovering Catholic. I was raised in the Catholic faith but I am very spiritualistic and I got in touch with my own spiritual beliefs, which took a great deal of searching, personal work, and a great deal of healing." Likewise, Simon identified himself as a Catholic but later on in the interview told me: "It's the balance, it's the harmony. I've become a fundamentalist Taoist I guess. I just feel that things are going to come up but I don't fight things either. I liken myself to a stick or a log floating down a river." Lindsay's agnosticism includes a smattering of several religious belief systems.

> Well, mind and spirit in the sense that I believe a lot of Oriental philosophy of really seeking within your self and being really quiet and balanced within yourself. I have a belief that there are people out there who have a higher power than ours. I don't believe that one person created the universe. I wouldn't say that I'm an atheist; I may be slightly agnostic.

Some of these informants saw a relationship between their spirituality and their use of alternative health care. For example, Jane told me: "I'm into a lot of other things like spirituality that's not mainstream minded, so this [alternative therapy] is just part and parcel of the package." And Grace said: "My father was from a Mennonite background and we did try things that weren't tradition." However, while participation in alternative spirituality may predispose one to explore alternative therapies, using alternative approaches to health and healing does not necessarily imply participation in alternative spirituality. Sharma (1992:45) makes the same point more generally, concluding that "using 'alternative' medicine ... is not necessarily associated with adherence to an 'alternative' culture or lifestyle, but some cultural and recreational activities are more likely than others to channel information about non-orthodox medicine."

The Canadian Medical Association concludes that there is nothing distinguishing about the population of users of alternative therapies; rather, they are representative of the general population (CMAJ 1991).[7] Similarly, Sharma (1990:128) contends that "users come from a wide range of backgrounds." This holds true for the people who participated in this research. There was little if any variation by sex, age, ethnic category, or SES—neither in terms of accessing alternative therapies, of beliefs about alternative approaches to health and healing, nor of the impact participation in alternative health care had on informants. Rather, the user of alternative therapies is no different from any other person engaged in health-seeking behaviour, and arguments that those who participate in alternative forms of health care are particular types of people remain unconvincing.

NOTES

1. Portions of this chapter were originally published in the journal *Complementary Therapies in Medicine* (2001), 9:105–110.
2. See also Anyinam (1990); Eisenberg et al. (1993, 1998); Jingfeng (1987); Montbriand and Laing (1991); Murray and Rubel (1992); O'Connor (1995); and Taylor (1984).
3. See Achilles et al. (1999); Eisenberg et al.(1993); Fulder and Munro (1985); Furnham and Bhagrath (1993); Kronenfeld and Wasner (1982); McGuire and Kantor (1987); Moore et al. (1985); Murray and Shepherd (1993); O'Connor (1995); Pawluch et al. (1994, 1998b); Ramsay et al. (1999); Sharma (1992); and Thomas et al. (1991).
4. See also de Bruyn (2001); Glik (1988); Murray and Shepherd (1993); Sharma (1992); Vincent and Furnham (1996); and Wellman (1995).
5. This sub-sample consisted of two hundred and eight respondents who used alternative therapies in the six months prior to the survey, who did not discuss their alternative therapy use with their doctors, and who responded to the question: "If you were to tell your doctor about using these alternative health services (not including chiropractor) do you think your doctor would say that they would...?" Response categories included: help you, not help you, make little difference to your health, and don't know. (Canada Health Monitor 1993:149, table 45b).
6. It is a matter of considerable debate whether this is due to a greater incidence of morbidity among women than among men, or to the more frequent medicalization of women's bodies and lives (Miller and Findlay 1994).
7. See also Coulter (1985); Donnelly et al. (1985); Furnham and Munro (1985); Furnham and Smith (1988) Kronenfeld and Wasner (1982); and Northcott (1994).

CHAPTER TWO

How People Use Alternative Therapies

While the user of alternative therapies is no different from any other health seeker, the way in which those who spoke with me experience using alternative therapies is a distinct process dependent on developing ever-expanding alternative health care networks composed of alternative therapies and the people who use them (de Bruyn 2001). Creating these networks is rarely accomplished in a systematic fashion; rather, it is a matter of one thing leading to another (Glik 1988; Sharma 1990). For example, Pam told me, "I picked up a couple of books and sort of one thing has led to another. From reading one book I get reference to another book"; and Natalie said, "Well I started off with positive thinking books, from there I went to tapes on healing and then I started taking courses on therapeutic touch and went from therapeutic touch to the results system."

For many informants, one thing leading to another involved serendipitous encounters with key individuals (Deierlein 1994). For example, Greg just happened to run into his brother-in-law, who is a naturopath:

> I caught some kind of stomach bug or whatever, and I'm staggering back across the street with a little prescription from my doctor and I happened to walk past my brother-in-law, and he could see that I was pretty wobbly, and he looked at the prescription and he figured the whole idea was just to shut the whole body down. He said: 'Come on into my office.'

Similarly, when I asked Natalie how she had found her healer, she described the key encounter which led her to explore alternative health care:

> I was going food shopping and my car went to the right when it was sup-posed to go straight, so I said: 'Okay, car, take me to where you want me to go.' Then all of a sudden there's a great big sign saying psychic fair, so I went

in. I said: 'I'm supposed to see someone here but I have no idea who.' I don't know why I just knew I had to see a psychic.... She's the one that said she was going to a healer in Quebec and she said: 'You've gotta go.'

Those informants who espoused non-mainstream spiritual philosophies tended to attribute these encounters to destiny or fate. According to Lorraine,

One girlfriend said: 'This doctor's speaking on natural medicine, would you like to go?' So I said yes, but that night there was a snowstorm, so can't go. Then her name [came] up again about three times and I thought, well destiny is telling me go to this doctor and finally I got to go to her. I do believe that it's part of your predestined path to get into this kind of thing.

In like manner, Trudy associated these encounters with the inscrutable workings of the universe:

I also believe, and have experienced, that usually whatever it is you're looking for, the people and the circumstances sort of fall into place, even if you don't know what it is. You just discover it.... If you're focussed on something all the pieces come. You just have to do your part and the universe takes care of the rest.

No matter how they make sense of these key encounters, one thing leading to another results in the development of ever-expanding networks of users and sources of alternative health care. In Laura's words:

I work part-time for a little store and a customer came in who I know and she was lamenting that her one son had just been diagnosed as having this wheat allergy and she said: 'And he's got a birthday party on Saturday and I don't know what to do.' So I said: 'Call me tonight and I'll give you some places to go to and some ideas.' She phoned me a few weeks later and she said: 'Here's a recipe book that I've picked up that's really good.' So we've been swapping back and forth like that. Neighbour down the road was at work and somebody was lamenting her daughter is wheat sensitive now and this woman phoned me clear out of the blue. I think I've talked to maybe four people who have just called because somebody has been talking about a friend of a friend and so we've been networking.

Scott told me his network began with friends he met while at university:

> I started to use natural medicines like Echinacea and golden seal and mega-dosing on vitamin C. It was through friends of mine at school who just knew about stuff. Like they'd educated themselves or had known people and so forth. It was all through a network of friends basically that I got started.

These alternative health care networks were conceptualized in a variety of different ways by the people who spoke with me. For example, Natalie conceptualized this web of people as a grapevine: "I went to a healing circle. They'd hear about it through the grapevine, just people in conversation. Someone will overhear a conversation and say: 'My husband's got cancer' and someone will say: 'Oh I know a healing group.'" Betty likened these networks to an ever-expanding snowball:

> Once you start in this field it's amazing the people you run into that are also interested, the places you get invited to. 'Hey there's a course on so and so; are you interested?' You just keep going and the snowball just keeps getting bigger and bigger.

Finally, Lorraine used the analogy of the Internet. She told me: "Guest speakers would come and lecture on all of these different topics so therefore you meet this person, this person, this person, 'Well I'm interested in this,' 'Well go and see this person.' It's like an Internet of people."

ALTERNATIVE HEALTH CARE NETWORKS

Wellman (1995:234) points out that; "as people go about their lives, they receive information from a variety of sources," and the Canada Health Monitor (1993) found that 24 percent of respondents learned about alternative therapies[1] through the means of common knowledge. Similarly, the people who participated in this research achieved *entrée* into alternative health care in a variety of largely informal ways. The alternative health care networks these people describe are made up of friends and acquaintances, family members who use alternative therapies, print media, specialty and mainstream retail venues, service organization and other institutions, alternative practitioners and holistic health centres, allopathic physicians, and the work place.

Friends

People most frequently discover alternative therapies through friendships (de Bruyn 2001; Fulder and Munro 1985; Hedley 1992; Moore et al. 1985; Sharma 1990, 1992). For example, the Canada Health Monitor (1993) reports that of those Canadians surveyed[2], almost half had done so on the recommendation of friends. It is therefore not surprising that the people who participated in this research most often found out about alternative therapies through friends and acquaintances. For instance, Scott told me, "I met this [practitioner], it was actually through her daughter who was a friend of mine"; and Lorraine said, "I went with [a friend] to her [naturopathic] doctor this one time and I sat in on one session with her and I quite liked what I saw, so I decided that I wanted to have my own." Similarly, Nora found out about homeopathy through friends who were her neighbours:

> My friend, she and her husband lived on the fifth floor in the late 70s, early 80s, and he had a lot of chronic skin problems. She went down to one of the natural food stores and came back with a homeopathic remedy and that was my introduction to it.

Some informants also had friends who were alternative practitioners themselves. For instance, Grace told me, "The woman that I go to has been a friend. I had known her before she became a naturopath." Wellman (1995:225) argues that people are most likely to access alternative therapies through what she calls "weak-ties," such as friends of friends rather than close friends or family members. However, at least where initial contact is concerned, the people who participated in this research most often first tried alternative therapies on the recommendation of people they considered friends rather than acquaintances.

The Media

The second most popular gateway to alternative health care for the people who took part in this research was print media, specifically books, newspapers, and posted notices. For Natalie, self-help books were her point of access: "I started off with positive thinking books, then I went to Shirley MacLaine's books and that really got me thinking there's something else out there. I read books constantly on healing, healing with the hands, healing with the mind and spirit." Others were reading or collecting books for a purpose they didn't originally see as directly related to health care. For example, Roger sought out alternative therapies after reading a book on running:

> I just went to a weekend workshop after reading a book by Moshe Feldenkrais.... Actually it was a book on running about sort of contemporary approaches to training, development of flexibility and all this sort of stuff. The Feldenkrais method was described in greatly superlative terms so I thought, well, that's interesting, and then I read a book by Moshe and I just went from there. So it was really more through the running originally than through a therapy, alternative medicine frame of reference.... Anyway, that was my first *entrée* into anything that is now in any way related to alternative medicine.

Once having become involved in using alternative therapies, these people began collecting books on alternative health and healing. This was the case for Laura:

> I have a library of books, they're at my beck and call in the middle of the night and on weekends when naturopaths don't tend to be.... If I can't find the information in my book I call my girlfriend who has different books. We tend to buy different books so that we have that ability to do that.

Similarly, Randal told me:

> I would read through every book. I'm not a reader generally: give me a novel and it will take me forever to read, give me a book on herbology and I've got it gobbled up in a night because it gonna keep me alive. It's the food of life, it's the knowledge of life, exploring that and how not to tox-ify myself with it.

Other types of media also play a role in an individual's use of alternative health care (Donnelly et al. 1985; Moore et al. 1985). For example, the Canada Health Monitor (1993:142) found that 18 percent of respondents accessed alternative therapies through the "media (newspaper, radio, TV, etc.)." For instance, Simon said: "I guess the media has a part to play in it whether it's through the radio or TV, science programs, magazines, newspapers. Actually I have a scrapbook of newspaper articles"; and while Laura initially attempted to find a midwife through friends and acquaintances, it wasn't until she saw a notice posted in a bookstore that she was successful. In Laura's words:

> I basically started from scratch and asked everybody I could think of who might possibly know and I went to the Women's Book Store[3] and there was some information there about a woman who provided labour support. I called her and she recommended a few midwives and I called them.

The literature is somewhat inconsistent as to the importance of print and other media in facilitating access to alternative therapies. On the one hand, Fulder (1996) argues that the role they play is minimal. On the other are Glik's (1988) and Sharma's (1992) more persuasive assertions that people often come to use alternative health care via the media. For instance, Anyinam (1990:72) writes that in Canada, "[a] plethora of books, news reports, and T.V. programs have ... tended to increase interest in alternative medicine" and, as demonstrated, print media played an instrumental role in gaining access to alternative health care for the people who took part in this research. Yet, none of the people who spoke with me said they gained access to alternative therapies through information obtained via the Internet. This is no doubt partially due to the fact that the majority of people I interviewed were between forty-one and fifty-nine years of age and therefore less likely than individuals in their 20s and 30s to regularly use the Internet as a source of information. However, given the "exponential growth of information about complementary therapies which is available in all popular media," including the Internet, the role of the Internet in how people use alternative health care should not be discounted (Achilles et al. 1999:269).

Family

Several of the people I spoke with first tried alternative therapies on the recommendation of family members. For example, Marie told me, "I have a niece who has always been into alternative therapies and she said: 'Why don't you try some of the remedies that are out there?'" Similarly, Hanna's then father-in-law introduced her to yoga:

My ex-husband's father had bronchitis and he used to do these breathing exercises. And when I was about seventeen or eighteen I would just sit and watch him in the chair doing specific breathing, and I asked him what it was and he said it was yoga breathing. I asked him all about it.

Greg was also introduced to alternative health care by a family member, one who happened to be an alternative practitioner himself. According to Greg, "The way I got involved was because my ex-wife's brother was a chiropractor who was starting to get into naturopathy." While family members, spouses, and/or partners were important to these people in initially accessing alternative therapies, consistent with Wellman's (1995:225) arguments that recommendations to use alternative therapies come for people with whom one has "weak-ties," family members did not play a significant role in their continued negotiation of alternative health care networks.

Commercial Outlets

Another important part of these informants' alternative health care networks is commercial outlets (de Bruyn 2001; Glik 1988). Several of the people who spoke with me patronized stores that specialized in the sale of alternative remedies. For instance, Nora told me, "[We] discovered [a] homeopathic store which is this wonderful place that's right out of Dickens." In contrast to the Canada Health Monitor's (1993) finding that only 7 percent of their respondents learned about alternative therapies through health food stores, several of these informants accessed alternative remedies through natural or health food stores. For example, Laura believes that "They're a really good source of information. If you just go in there and ask, they can pretty much tell you where to find the answers or give them to you." Others located information on alternative therapies by frequenting new age or other specialty bookstores. According to Scott, "I found that group through a bookstore. They sell all kinds of things from Tibet and there was a poster and I called the guy up and we arranged an interview." Laura, has also found a variety of books on alternative therapies through a major chain of popular bookstores. She said: "I was really impressed with their alternative section. It seemed just as well stocked as any other section." Finally, some of the people who participated in this research told me they had seen alternative remedies for sale in pharmacies. In Nora's words, "A lot of these preparations are more commercially available, i.e., drugstores."

That information about alternative therapies is available in mainstream bookstores is an indication of the growing popularity of alternative health care in Canada as well as the revenue such popularity can generate for retail establishments. Furthermore, that alternative remedies are stocked in pharmacies reflects the continued co-option of alternative therapeutic modalities by the medical community (Saks 1998).

Public and Private Institutions

A variety of public and private institutions serve as access points to alternative therapies (Pawluch et al. 1998b; Mason 1993). In Hanna's case, the point of *entrée* was the public library: "When I was eighteen I went to the local library and there was a yoga teacher there." A number of educational institutions also offer seminars, workshops, and courses featuring alternative health care (Glik 1988; Sharma 1992). For instance, the Canada Health Monitor (1993) found that 25 percent of Canadians surveyed learned about alternative therapies through educational institutions. Roger, for example, discovered the healing potential of meditation through a continuing education course: "I just happened to see an evening course in meditation was being offered and I thought well, I had a taste of that some years ago, I think I'll just go and jump in and find out more about it." Finally, a variety of service organizations and voluntary associations provide information about alternative health care. For example, in a report for the Canadian AIDS Society, Mason (1993) found that 31 percent of those surveyed responded that their primary sources of information about alternative therapies were AIDS service organizations. As Randal informed me, "Within the AIDS committees, they have a list of all the natural therapies, whether it be *reiki*, therapeutic touch, laying on of hands, massage, reflexology, acupuncture."

Alternative Practitioners and Alternative Health Centres

As one would expect, contact with one alternative practitioner can direct people to other alternative therapists (Wellman 1995). For example, a conversation with a *reiki* practitioner led Lucy to a chiropractor. She said:

> I went down and found the person who is now the director of the Wellness Centre and went in and told him that I had a pinched nerve or whatever,

and he told me that he really wasn't familiar with that aspect, but that he knew that my back was out of order because my head was not equalizing properly down the rest of the body. First of all he recommended a chiropractor to get that part straightened away and then go from there.

In addition, Hedley (1992) argues that people are able to access alternative therapies through an increasing number of professional services and holistic health centres. Surprisingly, however, only a few informants found alternative therapies through holistic health centres. In Marie's words:

Then I heard about the Wellness Centre.... I talked to a couple of the therapists at the Wellness Centre and a few other people I know, massage therapists, aromatherapists, *shiatsu* therapists, acupuncture, to see which route I was going to go with this and I had decided to go with acupuncture.

Allopaths

The Canada Health Monitor (1993) found that 23 percent of the people they surveyed were directed to alternative therapies by an allopathic physician. Likewise, a similar proportion of the people who spoke with me found their way to alternative practitioners on the recommendation of an allopath. For example, Pam's doctor suggested she see a naturopath. She told me, "We have a friend, a doctor, we wanted her opinion and she said 'have a paediatric assessment done and an allergy assessment.' That's where we went to him [the naturopath]; he was recommended by my GP." Furthermore, almost as many informants accessed other alternative therapies and/or practitioners through allopaths as through alternative practitioners. This is somewhat surprising, as people remain reluctant to disclose their use of alternative therapies to physicians (Eisenberg et al.1993; Montbriand and Laing 1991; Perlman et al. 1999; Ramsay et al. 1999). However, to the degree that the boundaries between allopathic and alternative health care continue to blur (Northcott 1994; Tataryn and Verhoef 2001), and physicians become more knowledgeable about alternative therapies, these types of referrals are likely to become more common.

Non-Mainstream Spiritual Groups

A less common initial access point to alternative health care for these informants is membership in a non-mainstream spiritual group. For

porous, they only envision movement across the boundaries between the folk and professional spheres and those between the folk and popular sectors. Furthermore, Sharma (1993:16) charges that they fail to fully explain how "healing practices may shift their location from one sector to another" and that they do not account for "professionalization as a dynamic process in 'alternative' medicine in the West." In contrast, a more accurate rendering of the health care system would conceive of boundaries that are permeable between each of the sectors within the system. Thus, not only would individuals who self-treat with alternative therapies and who later decide to seek training to practice them, move from the popular sector to the folk sector; depending on the type of training they receive, they may also move from the popular sector into the professional sphere. Take for example the case of the person using homeopathic remedies as part of his or her own personal health care regimes. If this individual later seeks training as a naturopath at the Canadian College of Naturopathic Medicine, he or she would move into the professional sphere. In contrast, if this individual apprentices with a non-regulated homeopathist, or is self-taught, he or she would move into the folk sector. Also problematic is that Chrisman and Kleinman's (1983) model isolates alternative practitioners in the folk sector. In contrast, the therapies used and practised by the people I spoke with can exist in all three of the spheres of the health care system. For instance, alternative therapies are often practised by those Chrisman and Kleinman (1983) would place in the professional sector, such as nurses who use healing touch in hospitals. Thus, rather than making distinctions based on types of therapies, the only fruitful distinction to be made between the sectors of the health care system is whether or not the individuals within them are regulated in some fashion (Saks 1997b). Finally, Chrisman and Kleinman's (1983) model does not account for the difficulty in accessing alternative health care experienced by lay people, including many of the people who participated in this research (Achilles et al. 1999; de Bruyn 2001; Low 2001b; Pawluch et al. 1998b).

What better reflects the health-seeking experiences of the people who participated in this research, as well as the position of alternative therapies within the health care system, is the following model (see Figure 2.1 on next page). Similar to Chrisman and Kleinman's (1983) popular sector, I include in the lay sector those activities people take on their own—in interaction with family members, through friendship networks, and/or within the larger community—to care for their health. In the lay sector, for instance,

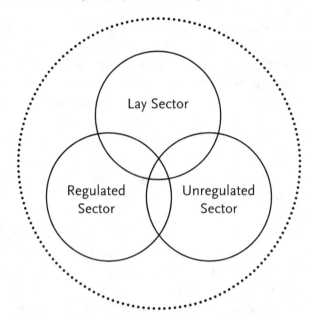

Figure 2.1. The Health Care System

the individual may self-treat, as Chrisman and Kleinman (1983:571) note, by using "patent medicines, prescription medicines which have been obtained from practitioners, ... pharmacies, ... or from family and friends." However, they may also self-treat by buying a homeopathic remedy in a grocery store, or by self-diagnosing a weakened immune system for which they compensate by taking vitamin C or garlic capsules. Moreover, what Chrisman and Kleinman (1983) call the folk sector is better conceptualized as the unregulated sector. Within this sphere one would find individuals who identify themselves as healers or practitioners but who are not regulated by legislation or who do not operate under the auspices of socially legitimated, professional associations. For instance, individuals who practice *reiki* out of their homes or a physician who uses alternative therapies not officially sanctioned by professional bodies such as the Canadian Medical Association. In the regulated sector I include health care practitioners governed by legislation and/or regulated by professional associations. Here we find chiropractors, naturopaths, and midwives in addition to allopathic health care professionals. The other substantial change I make to Chrisman and Kleinman's (1983) model is to encircle the three spheres of the health care system by a boundary. This perimeter is represented by a dotted line to indicate that access to any form of health care can be more or less limited in any given place, at any given time, to any given person; for instance, someone who can not find a family doctor, or who is on a waiting list for specialty medical services such as MRIs, or who would like to use acupuncture to cope with chronic pain but is unable to locate a practitioner.

In sum, accessing alternative therapies means finding a point of *entrée* into the alternative healing networks within the larger health care system. Once *entrée* is achieved, using alternative therapies is a matter of negotiating an infinite number and variety of alternative health care networks. For the people who participated in this research, negotiating these networks was experienced as a long, incremental process. According to Roger,

> It was over a long period of time. It's one of these incremental things. I had read things about the use of Chinese herbal medicine also in the past few years in connection with the chronic fatigue syndrome. I had a friend in the training who was very involved in that, so I learned a little bit about it in a very superficial way. Not personally too interested at the time, but it's sort of filed away there. I decided that I would investigate; I guess it was through a friend of mine partly, even though I'd done reading, like I said earlier. She had highly recommended this person, a doctor from China, that this doctor had been helpful for a friend of hers who had problems with these things; so I decided to go.

Most conceptualized this ongoing process as a search or journey: "I would say that was the beginning of a sort of over-all healing journey that I've been on" (Scott). "I was looking for my healing. It was my own search for my own healing" (Trudy). "In August I had a series of events, that's basically when I started searching for ways of healing myself" (Brenda). What distinguishes this long, incremental process from general health-seeking behaviour, and makes it truly alternative for these informants, is that in participating in alternative health care, in interaction with alternative practitioners and other lay users of alternative therapies, these people began to espouse alternative ideologies of health and healing.

NOTES

1. With the exception of chiropractic treatment.
2. Those who had consulted an alternative practitioner in the six months prior to the survey.
3. The Women's Book Store is a pseudonym.

CHAPTER THREE

Why People Turn to Alternative Therapies

The majority of researchers investigating why people seek out alternative approaches to health and healing have been concerned with discovering the motivating factors for individuals' use of alternative health care. Some authors argue that participation in alternative therapies represents an overall disenchantment with biomedicine (Furnham and Kirkcaldy 1996).[1] Others contend that people are drawn to alternative therapies, not so much out of a dismissal of allopathic care, but because they are attracted to aspects of alternative health ideology, such as desire for control over health and healing (Yates et al. 1993)[2] or a belief in a holistic approach to health care (Murray and Shepherd 1993).[3] Finally, Vincent and Furnham (1996) conclude that it is both dissatisfaction with allopathic health care and the appeal of alternative therapies that drive people away from biomedicine and towards alternative health care. These contrasting views have been conceptualized as the push/pull debate by Furnham and Smith (1988), among others (Vincent and Furnham 1996; Kelner and Wellman 1997; Sharma 1990). The question becomes: Are people pushed away from allopathic medicine and, as a consequence, pushed towards alternative therapies, or are they pulled towards alternative health care and, consequently, pulled away from allopathic medicine?

However, the explanations for why people turn to alternative health care subsumed within the push/pull debate are problematic for a number of reasons, not the least of which is that what are commonly reported in the literature as motivating factors in people's use of these therapies did not figure prominently amongst the people who participated in this research. In general, the people who spoke with me did not turn to alternative therapies for ideological reasons; they were neither seeking a holistic approach to health and health care, nor seeking control over matters of health and healing. Nor does dissatisfaction with allopathic medicine alone sufficiently explain why these people first engaged in alternative approaches to health and healing. Rather, in participating in alternative therapies, they were actively seeking relief from problems for which they found little or no redress in other quarters.[4]

MOTIVATING FACTORS

The various reasons cited in the literature for people's decisions to use alternative therapies can be grouped into two categories: those relating to ideological aspects of alternative approaches to health care and those concerning dissatisfaction with allopathic medicine. However, the people who took part in this research rarely identified ideological issues as reasons for their decisions to first seek out alternatives. While these informants made reference throughout their interviews to a variety of ideological components of the alternative model of health and healing they espouse, including a belief in the value of a holistic approach to health care or therapies that allow them to take control of health and healing, these beliefs were almost never voiced in conjunction with the accounts they gave of why they first turned to alternative therapies. Furthermore, while dissatisfaction with allopathic medicine was mentioned by informants as concomitant with their initial participation in alternative forms of health care, it proves problematic to attempt to explain an individual's use of these therapies solely through a dissatisfaction with allopathic medicine.

Control

That alternative therapies allow individuals a greater degree of control over their health and health care is often specified as a motivating factor in people's participation in these therapies (Furnham and Beard 1995).[5] While the desire for control was certainly something the people I spoke with valued about alternative approaches to health and health care, when they spoke about why they first got involved in using these therapies, only one person, Laura, identified a desire for control as the issue prompting her to seek out alternatives therapies: "My midwife, she interviewed me and one of the first things she asked was why I wanted a home birth and I said: 'because the control thing was really big.'" For the rest of these informants, the possible benefits to be derived from taking control and being in control of one's health and health care were things they discovered through their on-going experiences with alternative therapies and, in particular, in interaction with alternative practitioners (Deierlein 1994)—in other words, after they first began using alternative forms of health care. For example, in talking about her encounters with her naturopath, Grace said, "She encouraged me to take control. So I decided I was going to go more into the alternative medicines. I stopped the massive amounts of drugs I was taking."

Holism

Another aspect of alternative ideology, holism, is said to be an important factor in people's choice of alternative approaches to health care (Murray and Shepherd 1993).[6] However, only two out of the twenty-one inform-ants referred to a desire for a holistic approach to health and healing as something motivating them to first seek out alternative therapies. For instance, Trudy was one of the two who indicated that her interest in holism predated her initial foray into alternative approaches to health and healing:

> I had a bladder infection and I knew that there was more to it. I realised that there was a lot more to it in terms of the whole psychology. I could understand that my body was responding to my own thinking and I was responding to my environment with my thinking. I came from a family of alcoholics, so I was also looking for my healing, so I got involved with the Wellness Centre.

Again, it was only through their experiences with these therapies, and in interaction with alternative practitioners, that the vast majority of these informants came to espouse alternative ideologies, including a belief in holism. For example, it was long after he first participated in alternative therapies that Greg began learning about alternative ideology from his practitioners: "They [practitioners] try and I listen and it's kind of, well it's [their] show and I'm not going to tell [them] how to conduct the symphony. *Yin* and *yang* and that whole thing. I'd be curious to read more about it." Clearly, the allure of alternative health and healing ideology was not the initial motivator for use of alternative therapies for nineteen of these twenty-one informants. However, these informants did identify dissatisfaction with allopathic medicine as something concomitant with their decisions to turn to alternative health care.

Dissatisfaction

Many authors argue that people turn to alternative therapies because they have recognized the limitations of Western medicine and/or are, in general, dissatisfied with allopathic approaches to health care (Fulder 1996)[7]. Similarly, almost all of the people who participated in this study associated disillusionment with biomedicine with their first experiences of alternative therapies. In Hanna's words: "I found traditional [allopathic] therapy wasn't helping me at all." The dissatisfaction with medicine expressed by these people took many forms. For some a profoundly negative experience with biomedicine led them to look for alternatives. Below, Lindsay and Hanna describe incidents of what they saw as medical negligence, something which led them to turn away from allopathic approaches. In Lindsay's words,

> I had a really bad experience with [one doctor]. I had a really bad infection and what he found out was that I was retaining about five hundred CCs of urine. He said that I was probably going to end up living on antibiotics for the rest of my life because every time I turned around I'd get a bladder infection. [That] made me decide.

And Hanna told me,

> Well the car accident, the therapy was making it worse. I kept going to my family doctor and saying, 'It's not just in the muscles; I think it's the nerves.' For a year she didn't send me to a neurologist. All I kept having was one x-ray after x-ray and, well, there were no bones injured. She wouldn't believe me until I said there was something drastically wrong behind the left eye. One night I woke up, it felt like I had had a stroke. That's why I've lost a lot of faith in the [medical] system.

For most other informants, however, a sense of dissatisfaction with allopathic medicine was more all-encompassing and tended to be focussed on discontent with medical professionals on the one hand and/or dissatisfaction with medical therapy on the other. Several told me that their sense of dissatisfaction with Western medicine was related to what they saw as arrogant or uncaring attitudes displayed by physicians (Taylor 1984).[8] For instance, in relating an encounter with his urologist, Greg said,

His idea was that it was diabetes and he said: 'Sorry to tell you this but there's nothing that I can do for you.' He was like a high-end repair shop, and if he couldn't do the high-end repairs, then I was wasting his time. He gave me three strips of, they reminded me of clarinet reeds actually. He said: 'Just take them home, take them in the bathroom, urinate on them and if they go green you're, no red, no green.' He couldn't remember which colour was diabetes and I'm kinda thinking 'Oh god!' That's maybe where I bottomed out with conventional medicine.

Further, Phripp (1991) argues that some people seek out alternative therapies in order to have their problem seen as legitimate. Legitimacy is often at issue in cases of environmental illness, chronic fatigue syndrome, or other problems that "do not ... fit accepted [biomedical] diagnostic categories" (Schneirov and Geczik 1996:640). Similarly, another type of discontent voiced by these informants came from having to convince medical professionals that their illnesses were real. For example, Grace told me she felt her doctor did not believe her when she told him about the pain she was experiencing:

My doctor didn't believe that I was still having chronic pain. Because I now suffer from these wonderful things called chronic pain symptoms which [doctors] don't know a whole lot about. So it had to be mental and he sent me to see a therapist. [My naturopath] didn't think I was crazy and that was even more reassuring because I felt that I was valid. The medical profession didn't believe that I was valid, that I was really legitimate.

Dissatisfaction most often arose in connection to allopathic methods of treatment (Northcott 1994).9 In particular, informants raised questions about the suitability and efficacy of allopathic therapy. In addition they voiced concern over the potential iatrogenic effects of medical treatment (Illich 1975). For instance, many informants believed a biomedical approach was not suitable for the kind of problem they had and/or found that allopathic medicine could not help them with their problem. Witness the case of Grace: "One day out of desperation I thought, 'Well I've tried all the other quacks [doctors], I'm going down the tubes. What have I got to lose?' So I called [my friend the naturopath] up and I said: 'I've tried all the other quacks, I might as well try you now.'" Jane sought out alternative therapies when she felt allopathic approaches did not work fast enough:

I ruptured a disk in my back and the conventional methods were muscle relaxers and painkillers and 'Lay on the floor and don't move for three weeks or we'll put you in the hospital in traction.' And it just wasn't quick enough and I thought there had to be other ways. So I started going to chiropractors then and I've been going ever since.

Most common was the belief that allopathic health care was inappropriate to chronic conditions (Pawluch et al. 1994; Sharma 1990, 1992; Wellman 1995). For example, Roger and Lucy turned to alternative therapies in response to chronic health problems for which they found no relief in allopathic medicine. Roger put it this way: "The whole area of managing chronic illness in one's life comes to mind as kind of a departure from a Western medical framework." And Lucy told me this: "The medical field felt that the chronic fatigue had created the liver damage, but when I went to the naturopath they discovered that cortisone has about three pages of counter indications. The medical field, they didn't know what to do."

Finally, several informants' expressions of dissatisfaction were related to concern over side effects and/or invasive medical technology (Campion 1993; Murray and Rubel 1992; Murray and Shepherd 1993; Pawluch et al. 1998b; Sharma 1992; Vincent and Furnham 1996; Wellman 1995). Hanna, for example, found side effects from medication problematic:

Medications just don't agree with me anyway and they made my mind so sluggish that I decided to just come off all the medication they had put me on and I stopped the physio and I worked out my own exercise program and got more into the herbs and vitamins. It took me three years but I got well from there.

Lucy told me she sought out alternative therapies when she developed new health problems as a result of allopathic treatment:

I was put on an inhaler. It was a minute dosage of cortisone and they didn't think it would create any problems. I was on it for twenty months and over that period of time the cortisone lowered my resistance and my immune system to such a degree that it was incapable of functioning, so I was diagnosed with chronic fatigue syndrome and over the next five years I went through hell.

Laura turned away from allopathic approaches partially out of fear of side effects and of the invasive nature of medical technology:

> It worked for me during my pregnancy and it was a great alternative to having to use medications you really didn't want to take when you're pregnant. And so that continued when I was breast-feeding for the same reasons. It just worked and I had no side effects. It was probably that I had read too much before I got pregnant and in my early pregnancy about how unnecessary some of the procedures were and the potential harm they could cause to be comfortable with them.

As the data presented here show, dissatisfaction with allopathic medicine was certainly something that was concomitant with these informants' decisions to turn to alternative health care. However, discontent with biomedicine alone does not sufficiently explain why people first use alternative therapies, if for no other reason than disillusionment with allopathic medicine does not necessarily lead to participation in alternative approaches to health and healing and is, in addition, something often expressed by those who have never used alternative therapies. (Sharma 1992). So how then do we explain the individual's use of alternative health care?

INDIVIDUAL PROBLEMS, ALTERNATIVE SOLUTIONS

Campion (1993:282) makes the point that people seek out alternative therapies because they "want to feel better," and Pescosolido (1998:219) concludes that people "continue to ask advice and seek help from a wide variety of lay, professional and semiprofessional others until the situation is resolved." Similarly, almost all of the people who took part in these interviews turned to alternative therapies because they had a particular problem causing them distress that they wished to solve. According to Jenny, "Initially I think you're just going to see somebody looking for answers." Finding little or no relief in other quarters, they began looking for alternative solutions. The dilemma faced by more than half of these people took the form of a physical problem or crisis. "My main concern was I'd just like to get my body back on track," said Greg. For the rest, the problem or crisis was personal (emotional, psychological and/or spiritual) in nature. According to Scott, "I really began to confront my own sort of stuff like emotional issues, looking at my childhood. So I was starting to see some different [alternative] therapists."

I discuss the categories of physical and personal problems/crises separately, even though the alternative model of health these informants espouse is based on a belief in an inextricable connection between mind, body, and spirit. I do this in part for clarity of prose but primarily because of the very few informants who cited a belief in a mind, body, spirit connection as the reason they first tried alternative therapies. For almost all informants, an initial foray into alternative health care was an instance of practical action taken in order to solve what, at that time, they saw as relatively discrete problems.

Physical Problems

For the majority of these informants, attempting to solve a physical problem or reacting to a physical trauma was the reason they first sought out alternative therapies. For some, the problem was something they assessed as relatively minor. In Greg's words, "I guess my first experience in what I'd call full-blown alternative medicine would be [when] I caught some kind of stomach bug." For others the problem was something new that they had never before encountered. For example, Betty told me, "I ended up running into some physical problems, two very infected ears, something I'd never had before, and a rash." Other informants sought out alternative therapies for help in recuperating from more serious trauma to the body. For instance, Hanna said, "I didn't really take [alternative therapies] too seriously until I had an injury, a car accident," and Simon told me, "I was quite into athletics. After I burned out of that I had to recuperate. I started looking into alternatives." The remainder of these informants turned to alternative therapies to address chronic physical problems. According to Lucy, "I had all the problems of chronic fatigue syndrome plus I had gained fifty pounds, but the medical field, their answer was 'Well, your liver is damaged, yes, but you can survive quite nicely.' And I thought, 'I want to do more than survive: I want to enjoy.'"

Personal Problems

Almost as many informants told me that they first experimented with alternative therapies in order to cope with personal problems or crises. For Natalie the significant event was the breakdown of her marriage: "I was in such a rut, my marriage was going downhill and I couldn't pull out of it. And there were such negative vibes in my home that I decided that the only way that I could pull out of it was to get positive vibes in my mind." Brenda identified overwhelming stress at work as the point of personal crisis that led her to seek out alternative therapies:

> I guess it's called 'burnout' and that's basically when I started searching for ways of healing myself. I was very career-driven. I was working as a senior manager; it was a very stressful environment. By the time the second week of January rolled by I said to somebody: 'I feel like I've lived a whole year already.' Everything was just wearing me down and then one day I went down to a meeting and I just froze. I couldn't process a page. I just sort of clenched my teeth, waited through lunch, and ran away.

Scott's personal crisis involved the break-up of his family and the end of an intimate partnership: "That time that I was getting into [alternative therapies] was also the time of my family really disintegrating, and I was feeling really suicidal, and actually becoming suicidal. My relationship ended around this time."

While people turn to alternative therapies for a variety of reasons, I have found that focussing on particular motivating factors is not as useful as discovering the "generic social processes" involved in their participation in alternative health care (Prus 1997:xi–xii). This was made plain to me when I found that explanations reported in the literature as to why people seek out alternative forms of healing were not significant factors in motivating those I spoke with to first use these therapies. As I have demonstrated, concept-ualizing people's initial motivation to use alternative therapies in push/pull terms is problematic. For instance, all but two informants were not pulled towards alternative approaches to health care. They were not shopping for an ideology[10] when they first sought out alternative therapies. Holism and control, both aspects of their alternative ideology of health, were beliefs they came to value and espouse after they began participating in alternative health care. They were things they learned through interaction with alternative practitioners and other users of alternative approaches to health and healing, making them a product of, rather than motivator for, their use of these therapies (Deierlein 1994). Push/pull explanations obscure this significant temporal aspect. Thus, ideological factors are better employed in explaining why people continue to use alternative therapies.

Furthermore, the argument that people are pushed towards alternative therapies as a result of dissatisfaction with allopathic medicine does not sufficiently explain why people turn to alternative therapies. While those who participated in this research did associate disillusionment with allopathic medicine with their initial forays into alternative health care, none had wholly rejected allopathic medicine in favour alternative therapies. And as Sharma (1992:77) rightly points out, dissatisfaction with allopathic medicine can not fully explain an individual's decision to turn to alternative therapies, as discontent with Western medicine is "by no means confined to users of complementary medicine." Seeing individuals' initial decisions to seek out alternative therapies in push/pull terms turns attention away from what is really at issue for these informants, namely, finding some sort of solution to health problems. In this case they found an alternative solution in alternative approaches to health and healing.

THE WIDER SOCIO-CULTURAL CONTEXT

I have argued that these informants' initial use of alternative therapies is an instance of problem-solving reflective of generic social processes. But in what social context does this generic process of problem-solving take place? Or more precisely, is the choice of alternative therapy as a solution to problems of ill health reflective of larger socio-cultural change whereby alternative solutions constitute a new option in health-seeking behaviour?

In addressing this issue, authors have explained lay participation in alternative therapies by placing it within the context of larger socio-cultural changes in beliefs about health, illness, and the body, which include the following: disillusionment with medical science; lay demands for a larger share of control over health and healing; and a belief in holistic health care, where "health is more than a lack of disease ... [resting] on harmony of body, soul, mind, and emotion, and satisfactory relationships with other people and with society as a whole" (Crellin et al.1997; Coward 1989:43–4). However, when the frame of analysis is one of the problem-solving actions of individuals, the image which emerges is one of consistency rather than change. To illustrate, the ideological components of the alternative model of health espoused by these people are not new in any objective sense. Rather, as Crellin et al. (1997:44) note, "there is an intriguing continuity in many beliefs about health and illness" over time. Culturally speaking, these ideas about health and healing were always there (Archer 1988). For example, elements of these informants' notion of holism harkens back to Galen and the four humours school (Ziegler 1982). Accordingly, it is not that the elements of the ideology are necessarily new; rather, it is that these beliefs have now been taken up by these informants in order to articulate a model of health care they perceive as alternative therapy. These ideological components are cultural symbols, ultimately subjective in nature (Cohen 1985:15). Thus, the people with whom Pawluch et al. (1994, 1998b) spoke were able to use many of the same symbols, or elements of health ideology, to create a complementary rather than alternative solution to health problems.

Moreover, there has always been a plurality of healing options available to the individual (O'Connor 1995). For instance, in the 1663 volume of the diary of Samuel Pepys, we read of his attempts to solve his health problems by choosing between remedies offered by the apothecaries and those advocated by the doctors of physique (Latham and Mathews 1995). Likewise, Connor (1997:59) points out that it was only in the latter part of the nineteenth century that healing options were seen to narrow for Canadians:

> In addition to those practitioners who would be recognized as physicians by today's criteria ... there existed a smaller group of other medical practitioners ... includ[ing:] female midwives, commercial vendors of medicines, and domestic or lay healers; ... [and] sectarian practitioners.

The same phenomenon is evident in the British context, where "the evolving boundaries between orthodox and unorthodox medical knowledge ... can be highlighted with reference to the period of two or three centuries leading up to the first half of the nineteenth century" (Saks 1996:29). More to the point, the boundaries that emerged did not eradicate all forms of health care other than allopathic medicine; rather, they remained within the health care system (Bakx 1991), their ideological underpinnings part of the symbolic framework of "ideas which at any given time have holders," ready to be used by people in their efforts to solve health problems (Archer 1988:xix). Hypothetically, even if non-allopathic approaches to health care had been wiped out during this brief period, the individual always had the option of self-care or the option of doing nothing about his or her health problems.

Therefore, the nature of the actions of individuals in choosing this option can not be said to have changed; rather, they were, and remain, attempts at solving problems of ill health. On the other hand, what has changed is that there is now something people call alternative therapy, or complementary health care, or integrative medicine, the symbolic components of which have always been part of the ideology of health care options available to people in solving health problems. Conceptualizing health-seeking behaviour as a generic process of problem-solving allows us to account for whichever solution, alternative or otherwise, individuals choose.

While alternative health and healing ideology was not a significant factor in motivating the people I spoke with to begin using alternative health care, its importance should not be discounted, as these beliefs are something that individuals acquire through their participation in alternative health care and something that holds importance for them in their continued use of alternative therapies. Moreover, these ideologies form their alternative models of health and healing.

NOTES

1. See also Anyinam (1990); Fulder (1996); Furnham and Smith (1988); Monson (1995); Northcott (1994); and Taylor (1984).
2. See also Coward (1989); Dunfield (1996); Easthope (1993); Furnham and Beard (1995); Furnham and Bhagrath (1993); Murray and Rubel (1992); Northcott (1994); and Vincent and Furnham (1996).
3. See also Anyinam (1990); Dunfield (1996); Furnham and Bhagrath (1993); Northcott (1994); and Vincent and Furnham (1996).
4. It is important to note that no pattern emerged in the analysis between type of therapy used, or length of time using a therapy, and reasons informants gave as to why they first began using alternative forms of health care.
5. See also Coward (1989); Dunfield (1996); Easthope (1993); Furnham and Bhagrath (1993); Murray and Rubel (1992); Northcott (1994); Vincent and Furnham (1996); and Yates et al. (1993).
6. See also Anyinam (1990); Dunfield (1996); Furnham and Bhagrath (1993); Northcott (1994); and Vincent and Furnham (1996).
7. See also Anyinam (1990); Furnham and Smith (1988); Monson (1995); and Northcott (1994).
8. See also Anyinam (1990); Dunfield (1996); Easthope (1993); Fulder (1996); Furnham and Bhagrath (1993); Furnham and Smith (1988); Murray and Rubel (1992); Riley (1980); and Vincent and Furnham (1996).
9. See also Anyinam (1990); Coward (1989); Moore et al. (1985); Murray and Rubel (1992); Murray and Shepherd (1993); Sharma (1992); Taylor (1984); and Vincent and Furnham (1996).
10. I am grateful to Steven Crocker for this apt turn of phrase.

CHAPTER FOUR

An Alternative Model of Healing

While I have shown that there are very real problems in conceptualizing alternative healing residually by distinguishing it from biomedical treatment, residual means of definition proved very popular among the people who participated in this research.[1] When I asked Richard how he would define alternative healing, he said, "Alternative healing is anything that would not be considered the traditional [Western] approach to it." And Lindsay told me alternative therapy is: "Stuff that's out of the realm of typical Western medicine," which Brenda echoed with "I guess to me what alternative means is anything which is nonmedical." While Richard, Lindsay, and Brenda were among the few who stated it so explicitly, defining alternative healing by differentiating it from allopathic approaches was implicit throughout all the other interviews. The particular distinguishing criteria used by the people who participated in this research can be grouped into three broad categories: the focus and purpose of therapy, the nature of the client/practitioner relationship, and alternative healing techniques.

THE FOCUS AND PURPOSE OF THERAPY

The people who took part in this research used a series of alternative versus allopathic statements in explaining what they see as distinctive about the focus and purpose of alternative therapy. Some informants highlighted the general approach to health problems, for example holism; while others focussed on specific techniques they associated with alternative healing, such as natural remedies. What is common in all cases, however, is that they distinguish alternative therapy by differentiating it from what they see as the negative standard of Western biomedical treatment (see Figure 4.1).

Alternative vs. Allopathic	
Chronic	Acute
Holistic	Dualistic
Individualistic	Generic
Preventative	Curative
Natural	Chemical
Slow & Gentle	Fast & Brutal
Non-Invasive	Invasive

Figure 4.1. Alternative Versus Allopathic Healing

Chronic vs. Acute

All the people who spoke with me said that serious, acute, and emergency situations are the proper sphere of allopathic medicine. For example, Roger told me that while he is extremely reluctant to use allopathic therapies, he does feel that "medicine has some very powerful weapons" to mobilize in cases of acute illness. As Richard graphically put it: "If someone comes to you with their finger half cut off you don't give them herbs to make it grow back." And Scott said, "Obviously if I got a bullet in the head then I'd just go to the hospital. If I'm having a heart attack I want to go to an allopathic medical doctor." In contrast, the purpose of alternative healing is to address chronic health conditions, a finding noted in much of the research on alternative therapies (Fulder and Munro 1985; Montbriand and Laing 1991; Pawluch et al. 1994; Sharma 1990, 1992). For instance, Lindsay told me, "If I had a ruptured appendix I don't think I'd go see a naturopath, I think I'd probably be here at [the hospital]. But, you know, for long-term things alternative therapies really helped me." Similarly, Grace said, "If it's not acute, if I'm not in extreme pain, with the kidney stone I had to go to the hospital. However, if it's not an acute thing that requires emergency service, I will turn to my alternative health care."

Holistic vs. Dualistic

Holism is perhaps most often cited as a defining criterion of alternative approaches to healing (Lowenberg1992).[2] Likewise, almost all of the people who spoke with me said that alternative therapy is holistic in its attention to mind, body, and spirit, as opposed to allopathic medicine, which focuses solely on the body.[3] In Nora's words: "One has to engage or enlist the person's body and mind, and I personally would add spirit, into their healing. It's not someone saying: 'Here, take two aspirin, call me in the morning.'" According to Hanna, this means addressing the "whole person" rather than merely the physical manifestation of disease. In her words:

> A doctor can say, 'Okay, we've removed the cancer, we've healed that patient.' But all they've done is remove the cancer and the patient can still be quite ill and develop another cancer because they haven't been nurtured and they haven't been made a whole person again.

Similarly, for Jane, alternative healing means "treating all of the person" rather than just the symptoms of the disease. She put it this way:

> You can't just say we're going to treat your stomach without saying, 'Well why is it the stomach? Is it just the diet? Does this person have emotional problems or stresses on their shoulders that's causing this problem?' You have to know the whole person before you can treat any one part of the person.

Individualistic vs. Generic

According to Lowenberg (1992) a central parameter of alternative healing from the practitioner perspective is belief in the uniqueness of the individual versus the allopathic medical assumption of generic disease and treatment regimes (Mishler 1989). Thus a few informants mentioned that, in contrast to a biomedical understanding, within alternative healing symptoms vary from person to person. Furthermore, what works as a remedy for one person may not work for another. Lindsay explained it this way: "Finding out more of what of how a person works as opposed to everybody's symptoms mean the same thing, just giving everybody the same thing.... I think each person's a little bit different."

Preventative vs. Curative

For several of the people who took part in the interviews, alternative healing is preventative, versus allopathic healing, which is cure-oriented

(Deierlein 1994; McGuire and Kantor 1987; O'Connor 1995; Pawluch et al. 1994; Sharma 1990). Natalie, a practitioner as well as a user of alternative therapies, believes that "traditional medicine is definitely not preventative medicine; mine's more preventative." Lucy also felt a focus on preventative care distinguished alternative from allopathic approaches. In her words: "Hopefully you can prevent the disease from occurring. There are diseases today that are horrendous that medication does wonders for, but [doctors are] totally mystified in preventing." An attendant belief held by these people is that alternative practitioners are looking for the causes of health problems, versus allopathic practitioners who only consider symptoms (Schneirov and Geczik 1996; Sharma 1990, 1992). For example, Lindsay and Greg both believe that allopathic therapy treats symptoms rather than addressing the underlying cause of health problems. According to Lindsay, "The problem I have with Western medicine, they treat the symptoms, not the problem. Don't just treat the fact that the nerves are pinched; treat the fact that you can fix why it's being pinched. Don't just mask the symptom." And Greg told me that he "went back after a month and a half of the [medication] and [the doctor] said: 'So how's it going.' I said: 'Well, I still have a bad back but I don't really care or feel about anything.'"

Natural vs. Chemical

Most of these informants defined alternative healing by claiming that alternative therapies are natural, versus allopathic medicine, which is chemically produced (Pretorius 1993; Sharma 1992); or in Natalie's words, poisonous: "They push pills, and pills I do not like taking, except for the odd vitamin. I don't think there is anything you put into your body that's so poisonous like a pill. I think it will keep you alive, but that's all it's doing; it's not really healing." For Lorraine, natural healing is associated with spirituality: "I do believe that God puts, for every disease or upset, a remedy in a natural form. I don't mean that I'm averse to taking penicillin or anything, but if you can help it, I don't believe in taking chemicalized things, synthetics."

Slow and Gentle vs. Fast and Brutal

Several of these informants said that one difference between allopathic and alternative approaches is that alternative healing takes time, versus allopathic treatment, which produces quick results (Glik 1988). "Homeopathy takes a little longer sometimes," said Grace, and Lorraine argued that "The main thing that people must understand is that this is not a 'one, two, three month you're finished' situation. Natural healing is the whole body, not just this, this, and this we're correcting: it's total health." Furthermore, these people value the fact that alternative healing takes longer than allopathic healing, and several of them linked the speed of allopathic results with trauma to the body. In Nora's words, "I really do think that allopathic medicine is really slam bang. It's very fast but it can also be quite brutal in the effects it has."

Non-Invasive vs. Invasive

Most of the people who participated in this research said that alternative therapies are different from allopathic medicine because they are non-invasive (Coward 1989; Cant and Calnan 1991; Goldstein et al.1987; Sharma 1992). In telling me why she chose a midwife for the birth of her child, Laura said, "I wanted a home birth because I wanted to avoid unnecessary medical intervention during the labour and delivery." Likewise, in describing foot reflexology, Lucy told me this:

> It's a non-invasive treatment. What have you got to lose? If you're prepared to undergo the knife, and all the problems and complications that could happen, rather than looking at another method that may be able to prevent surgery, why would you not think about it?

These people also believe that the invasive nature of allopathic medical therapy puts them at risk of "clinical iatrogenesis" (Illich 1975:22). For example, more than half the people I spoke with were concerned about unpleasant and/or dangerous side effects caused by medication (Monson 1995; Pawluch et al. 1998a; Vincent and Furnham 1996). In Laura's words, "Garlic and vitamin C may not work as well as an antibiotic, but it works enough to justify its use and it doesn't have the side effects." Some informants told me they felt allopathic medication caused them to develop additional health problems. "I've seen too many people who've gone through on antibiotics," said Lindsay. "They get loaded with these anti-biotics and then their body is open to everything." Some were concerned about becoming addicted to allopathic medications (Sharma 1990).

According to Marie, "It was very hard getting off the muscle relaxants, the codeine, the over-the-counter pain medication. It took actually over a year to get through all of that. It was quite a struggle." Others, like Jane, were concerned about having to take medication forever:

> I'm still not on blood pressure medication. I've had high blood pressure for five years now, because anyone I know who has gone on the medication, you never come off of it. Some people when they come off the pills, boom: they've had a stroke or a heart attack because the body can't regulate itself without that medication any more.

In contrast to the dangers they felt were inherent in allopathic medical treatment, these informants believe that alternative therapies are non-invasive, non-iatrogenic, and consequently safe to use, a belief mirrored in general lay perceptions of alternative approaches to healing (Boon et al. 1999; Boutin et al. 2000; Johnson 1999; Low 2001b). Grace put it this way: "What the ear candling can do, they go back to their doctor after it's been done and the ear's fine, or maybe just a little more cleaning needs to be done. It's gentler, it's safer, it's less traumatic." Similarly, Nora argued that, "There's nothing in homeopathy. You could take the whole rack and other than having a real lactose kind of over-reaction and sugar reaction, you know it's not going to harm you."

THE NATURE OF THE CLIENT/PRACTITIONER RELATIONSHIP

When informants spoke about the nature of the relationship between alternative practitioners and their clients, they did so by comparing it to, and distinguishing it from, what they saw as the typical doctor/patient relationship. In describing their encounters with alternative practitioners, they often began by giving an account of an unpleasant interaction with a physician, which they then contrasted with a positive depiction of their relationships with alternative practitioners. Simply put, what they value about alternative practitioners is that they are not medical doctors. The major distinguishing criteria they mentioned were attitude of the doctor or practitioner (Furnham and Bhagrath 1993), time spent with the patient or client (Cant and Calnan 1991),[4] and whether or not they feel their doctor or practitioner cares about them (Campion1993; Lowenberg 1992; Sharma 1992; Taylor 1984).

Attitude

Almost all of the people I spoke with told me that, in contrast to alternative practitioners, physicians are arrogant and/or condescending: "90 percent of the doctors, it's their way or no way" (Natalie) ; "The superciliousness of the manner of certain doctors. They were aloof, supercilious, pompous" (Jenny). Some, such as Hanna, said their doctors wouldn't listen to them:

> I went to see the doctor, then she sent me to a neurologist and there was a blood clot on the brain. But it had started to heal itself because it had been a few years since it happened. And because they really wouldn't listen at that time, there were a lot of things that could have helped that they didn't do.

On the other hand, these informants described their alternative practitioners as respectful and unpretentious. "They don't talk down to you," said Jane. "You might not know everything there is to know about this, but that's not because you're stupid or you're less educated; it's just there's so much out there. I find most alternative people do not display a superiority." Nor, as Laura explained to me, do they appear to be as preoccupied with professional boundary maintenance:

> When I went the first time and I said that I'd been to the doctor already, she wasn't threatened by that, whereas I felt that perhaps my doctor's reaction was one of feeling threatened. She never badmouthed doctors or said anything that made me feel that she was at all negative about conventional medicine.

Similarly, Nora linked the differences she saw in attitude between alternative practitioners and allopathic physicians to issues of professional power:

> Trying to talk to an allopathic medical person about medication, saying 'I prefer ampicillin because sulpha really has a bad effect on me. I prefer this dosage than this one.' They get just totally offended because you're on their turf; you're talking about medication and that's their business: they own it.

Furthermore, Lucy pointed out that, in her experience, alternative practitioners were more likely than allopathic physicians to admit that they are not omniscient: "I find the naturopaths are much more willing to say, 'I don't have the answer, I'll do research on it to find out what the answer is.' I don't ever think I've heard of a medical doctor saying 'I don't know, I'll do research.'"

Time

Most of the people who took part in this study distinguished between allopathic physicians and alternative practitioners on the basis of the amount of time spent with the patient or client. For example, Lucy and Grace both stressed that what is different about alternative practitioners is that they devote more time to consultation. Lucy put it this way: "They've got it timed that their visits are about ten minutes apart and you feel like you're in a factory. [Alternative practitioners] have an entirely different way of looking at it and one thing you find is that they listen and they take the time to question." Similarly, Grace said this:

> I had to take my naturopath's daughter-in-law over to her doctor one day and she was out in two minutes. When you go to see [a naturopath] you know you're going to be a little while because you have to go through all these symptoms. [The doctor] wasn't interested in any of that; he just wanted to write up a prescription. In and out; she was just a number.

Lorraine was the only informant who speculated that allopathic physicians' work loads constrain the amount of time they are able to spend with patients:

> As good as my doctor is, they're so busy now, it's just patient after patient after patient and I get the feeling that there's just not time for me to sit down and have a good talk with him. I never feel like that with [my naturopath]. Not that she doesn't have her patients booked on a regular basis, but you're going there once a month, which helps.

Caring

Finally, caring was another criterion many of these informants used in distinguishing between allopathic and alternative healing. Over half of them said that, unlike allopathic physicians, alternative practitioners sincerely care about their clients. Simon, who is an acupuncturist as well as a lay user of alternative therapies, put it this way: "Another difference between holistic practitioners and [allopathic] practitioners is they're in it for money, it's a profession. We're in it for our love of people." Caring also means attending to the client (Hare 1993; Monson 1995; Sharma 1992). In Jenny's words, "If you go for *reiki* or hypnotherapy you're getting the attention of somebody." Hanna, who practises yoga, spoke about caring and touching as hallmarks of alternative healing (Goldstein et al. 1987): "Caring is a major difference. The doctors don't have time or patience. People need time and care, and that heals more than anything. I show that I care and I touch and hug."

ALTERNATIVE HEALING TECHNIQUES

The people who participated in this research saw alternative healing techniques as informed by two key concepts: self-healing and healing energy. For these informants, self-healing comprises self-treatment, harnessing the body's ability to heal itself, and the power of the mind to effect healing.

Self-Healing

Most informants saw the ability to heal oneself as a major defining criteria of an alternative approach to healing (Furnham 1994; Lowenberg 1992).[5] Brenda put it this way: "Self-healing, the complexity of our bodies, the way it's all put together. And our minds, the complexity of our souls must be billions times greater. So I think only people themselves can truly heal themselves because of the complexity." Similarly, Marie told me this: "I had decided that it was time to get back to natural ways and looking inside for a lot of the answers to health questions, doing my own healing." For a few of these people, self-healing means to self-treat. As Laura said, "You can self-prescribe homeopathic remedies." However, for the majority of informants, self-healing involved using the body (Furnham and Bhagrath 1993; McGuire 1987) and the mind (Furnham and Kirkcaldy 1996; Lowenberg 1992) to effect healing.

For almost half of these people self-healing meant mobilizing the body's ability to heal itself. In Lindsay's words, alternative healing means "Do[ing] the stuff so you can let the body heal itself." And Scott said, "I think that homeopathic medicine can be very effective in bolstering your own body's process of trying to heal all the time." For some, this means maintaining and balancing a bodily system that is naturally designed to heal itself (Pretorius 1993). For example, in describing his experiences with massage therapy, Randal told me his therapist said, "I'm doing a massage on your lymphatic system. I'm draining out the toxins that are clogging it so your lymphatic system can deal with the disease a little bit better." Similarly, Greg said, "The idea of feeling better over all, and treating yourself well, and maintaining yourself, and giving your body a chance to do what it's able to do. You have to get your body up to a certain maintenance level so that it can do what it's naturally able to do." And Hanna told me this: "When you can, you then try and bring the body back into balance. And the only way you can really do that it by exercise and good nutrition to put the body into a situation where it can help itself."

For others, allowing the body to self-heal meant bolstering the immune system. For example, in talking about how she treats her husband's colds, Laura said, "I'll give him Echinacea or suggest he use some vitamin C or garlic to boost his immune system." Lindsay also believes in the value of strengthening the immune system to allow the body to heal itself: "I wanted to find if there was a way that I could strengthen my own body constitution so that it could fight off the infections more. So when I'm starting to feel sick, hopefully my immune system will kick whatever it is off sooner."

Self-healing also means using the power of the mind for healing. For instance, Lorraine said, "If you can get into this thinking pattern there's nothing that you can't heal in your own body," and Betty told me, "The human mind is a pretty powerful thing and I think even just with our mind alone, I think we can basically heal ourselves with our attitude or our thinking processes." Harnessing the power of the mind over the body to bring about healing can mean anything from general bodily maintenance through pain relief, to destroying tumours and cancerous cells. For instance, Jane visualized a video game character eliminating substances in the body not conducive to good health: "If I'm not feeling well when I go to bed, you know Pac Man? I just visualize it. I turn on my brain and I say: 'Okay, send them all out,' and they can chomp up anything in this body that's not good for it." Trudy also used visualization as a means of enabling the mind to engender healing:

> They had found early stages of cancer of the cervix and I believe, to this day, that if I had had more time to really work with it, that I would have been able to cure it without any kind of operation. I truly believe that,

and the reason why is because with visualization work, cancer is something that is in a physical spot, so it's easier to visualize on one spot and to do all the healing stuff on that one spot.

For Lindsay, using the mind to self-heal means having more of an overall awareness of her body rather than using visualization techniques: "I can be lying down and be having some muscle tightness or some pain and I feel like I can send my awareness down in my body to smooth out those muscles, and run it like a pulse of energy, and smooth them out as if there were hands smoothing them out, and I feel better." Finally, for Natalie, harnessing the power of the mind to heal requires faith: "I really think you can get rid of tumours. I think that you can open up you blood vessels if you have arterial sclerosis, but this takes a lot of believing in order for it to work."

Healing Energy

Almost half of the people who spoke with me said the use of healing energy as a therapeutic modality is a distinguishing characteristic of alternative approaches to healing. These informants told me that everything on earth, as well as in the universe, is composed of energy that can be mobilized to heal. "I believe," said Betty, "and so many others believe, that we can, well, everything's energy, all life is energy. I believe that you can give energy to others, you can actually send it to others." Similarly, Hanna said, "It's in the air that we breathe, it's energy, in the food that we eat, the vital life force. I've found that with yoga and reflexology and therapeutic touch, they all work, whether the person believes in them or not, because it comes from the practitioner trying to direct energy." For some of these informants, healing energy originates in the earth (Coward 1989; O'Connor 1995). For example, in describing how crystal therapy works, Jane told me, "It's drawing energy from the power within the earth and it's used for healing." Similarly, Lorraine said, "I use a lot of earth energy. I bring that up and pour it over the person. I ask mother earth to give us that. And a great part of all of this is acknowledging where these energies are coming from. I give thanks to mother earth for supporting us." For others, the source of healing energy is the universe of which all things are a part (Glik 1988; McGuire and Kantor 1987; O'Connor 1995). According to Marie, "*Reiki* is channelling of universal energy through hands to you, and you do with the energy what you need to do, wherever the healing needs to take place."

Finally, for others, healing energy has a spiritual dimension (Glik 1988; McGuire 1987; McGuire and Kantor 1987). In Jane's words, "Using the crystals for healing is spiritual. You have to believe that there's this power within these rocks and that the power comes from another source and it's a living thing, so that's a part of my spirituality." It is important to note that while I spoke to a variety of people from different age groups, religious backgrounds, educational backgrounds, and so on, I found very few relationships between *types* of people and beliefs about alternative healing. However, I did find a connection between participation in alternative spirituality and beliefs about a specific alternative healing technique. To be precise, it is not that people who participate in new age or non-mainstream spirituality are any more likely than those who do not to believe in the concept of healing energy. Rather, the distinction lies in what they believe to be the source of this energy. While most of the people who took part in this research believed in the concept of healing energy, informants who participated in new age or non-mainstream spirituality were more likely to believe the source of this energy to be metaphysical, originating in God, spirit, or the universe. In contrast, those informants espousing mainstream religious beliefs drew on scientific paradigms in attributing the origin of healing energy to the fact that the earth, and all things on it, are composed of energy.

In the end, these people define alternative healing by comparing it to, and differentiating it from, allopathic healing. In doing so they use a variety of distinguishing criteria comprising three broad categories: the focus and purpose of therapy, the nature of the client/practitioner relationship, and alternative healing techniques. While different informants focus on different distinguishing criteria, they all use allopathic medicine as their reference point in defining alternative healing. For example, whether or not an informant's emphasis is on attitude, caring, or time is not as important as the fact that what defines the nature of the alternative client/practitioner relationship is that it somehow differs from the negative standard of the doctor/patient relationship. Holism, a key component of these informants' alternative model of healing, also figures prominently in their alternative model of health. Like many concepts associated with alternative health care, holism is a complex, and at times ambiguous, term. In the following chapter I examine in more detail the concepts, including holism, that make up these informants' alternative model of health.

NOTES

1. However, this does not mean that these people see nothing distinct about alternative therapies, as is plain from the meaning they give to their model of alternative health. See chapter five for further discussion of this issue.

2. See also Dunfield (1996); Furnham and Bhagrath (1993); Furnham and Forey (1994); McGuire (1983); and Pawluch et al. (1994, 1998a).

3. See Saks (1997b) and Coward (1989) for a critical assessment of the argument that holism is exclusive to alternative health care.

4. See also Campion (1993); Fulder and Munro (1985); Furnham et al. (1995); Furnham and Forey (1994); Furnham and Smith (1988); Hare (1993); Sharma (1992); and Taylor (1984).

5. See also Fulder and Munro (1985); Furnham and Smith (1988); Glik (1988); Goldstein et al. (1987); McGuire (1987, 1988).

CHAPTER FIVE

An Alternative Model of Health

It is well established that there is no consensus as to how we should define concepts associated with alternative therapies. What is understood to be alternative health varies dependent on who is giving meaning to the concept and in which social context that definition occurs. However, this does not mean that we can not discuss alternative health; rather, what is necessary is that we specify in what context meaning is invoked (Low 2001). In this case, the model of alternative health I discuss below is based on the subjective perspectives of Canadian lay users of alternative therapies.

As I have demonstrated, the people who spoke with me sought out alternative health care to solve problems for which they found no redress in other quarters. While they were not shopping for an ideology when they initially explored alternative therapies, once they began participating in alternative approaches to health and healing, and through interaction with alternative practitioners and other users of alternative health care, they began to take on alternative ideologies of health. This belief system informs their alternative model of health, one that is made up of three conceptual categories: holism, balance, and control. Simply put, to be healthy is to be whole, which in turn is to be balanced, which in the end means being in, and subject to, control.

ALTERNATIVE HEALTH AS PROCESS

The people I spoke with see alternative health and alternative healing as concomitant ongoing processes. Health is not an achievable goal as such, but an ideal to which a lifelong healing journey takes one closer and closer. In other words, to be healthy is to be engaged in the process of healing. Some informants experienced this process as a quest. For example, Trudy said, "It was really more my own search for my own healing," and Randal put it this way:

"I started my five-year search for this sort of healing, something that I'm constantly going to be working at." Others likened the process to a pilgrimage: "I felt like I was on some kind of journey," said Scott, "some kind of a progression that had to do with looking at what was going on inside of me." In both cases the emphasis is on the process rather than the outcome. Nonetheless, these people do have a discernable model of health in mind, which they articulate through the conceptual categories of holism, balance, and control.

Holism

Holism is the concept perhaps most often associated with alternative therapies (Furnham and Smith 1988; Lowenberg 1992; McGuire and Kantor 1987; Pawluch et al. 1994). Accordingly, it came as no surprise when all but three informants said they believe that an alternative model of health is a holistic model of health. For instance, Nora told me that alternative health "means that the person, their body, is functioning really well, in a natural way. And that means that they have a kind of wholeness about them. Their whole being is integrated in some way and works together." But what does holism mean? Like many new age concepts, such as *wellness* or *centred*, the concept of holism is abstract and ambiguous. For instance, when I asked people to elaborate, most defined holism as the unity of mind, body, and spirit. Richard explained it this way: "Health is a state when you're in line with your spiritual, physical and mental, and you're pulling all your energies together." But what does unity of mind, body, and spirit mean? For these people it means being balanced.

Balance

Not only is alternative health a matter of the wholeness of the individual, but the person must also experience balance amongst the components of mind, body, and spirit (McGuire and Cantor 1987). Similarly, the people who participated in this research also emphasized the need for balance when discussing their beliefs about alternative health. For example, Trudy said, "I think ideally what well-being is, is a balance in heart, mind, body, and soul," and Jane told me that "Health to me is not just physical, it's mental and spiritual. If you're a truly well person then all those things need to be balanced." Likewise, Brenda provided me with a written autobiographical statement in which she stressed that balance is integral to alternative health: "I continue to explore opportunities specific to my own needs which will help me maintain the precious balance between mind, body, and spirit." But what does balance mean? For these informants, balance is made up of two concepts: balance in the body and balance in the self.

For almost half of the people who participated in this study, the concept of balance means balance within the bodily system. They said things such as, "My enzymes do change and you can tell when things start to get out of balance again" (Lucy); "If something happens you can re-balance yourself because there's so many different systems in your body that you can balance it" (Richard); and "Having a balance in the body, it does make sense in a way to me" (Greg). Under certain alternative ideologies of health, illness is said to arise when the flow of bodily energy is disharmonious or has been disrupted (Glik 1988; O'Connor 1995). Likewise, for some of these people, balance in the body also means the unblocked flow of energy throughout the body. These informants were most often those who were, or were in training to become, alternative practitioners. For example, in relating his understanding of how acupuncture achieves health, Simon told me this:

> Picture your body as a huge mansion: it's a temple; you open up certain windows in your house and get an air current through that's comfortable for you. You don't open all the windows because then doors start slamming. You open up strategic windows and you get the flow of air. Opening the windows to let the energy flow through at a better rate because it's sluggish, or I'll close off because it's too much energy.

Similarly, in telling me about *reiki*, one of the alternative therapies she uses, Marie said, "Get the body loosened up and then the emotion energy can start flowing. We're trained to feel where there are energy blocks in the body, where there's low energy or high energy." For most of the informants, however, the key to achieving balance in the body is awareness of, or listening to, the body. For instance, Lorraine used an analogy in explaining what listening to the body means: "Some very old cars are in very good condition, but you see a lot of new cars that are in very poor condition. It's the same with the body: it depends on the driver. Everything rests with the inner knowing, the spirit telling you what is right." Randal and Lindsay also stressed the intuitive skills necessary to listening to the body. According to Randal, "I don't feel strong enough necessarily to do a complete workout today, and that's just listening to my body [and saying to myself]: 'I think I'll take it easy today.' And every day it's always listening and monitoring." Lindsay had a similar view:

> People who get into some of the naturopathic things start to develop an awareness of their body and people that don't have that awareness don't believe it can actually happen. They don't believe that you can actually get in and feel yourself, and feel the inner harmony, and feel what's going on.

For others, being whole means that not only should the body be in balance, but one's self and one's life must be balanced as well. For example, in giving meaning to balance in the self, Jenny and Lindsay used analogies. According to Jenny,

> I see [being balanced] as being in the middle and being able to see all the sides around one as opposed to being on the edge of the same circle and you're just having to exercise all this energy just to stop from falling off. But if you're in the middle you can see everything around.

In contrast, Lindsay described being centred in the following way:

> If I'm centred I feel like I'm going forward. I can choose where I want to go, right, left, or straight. Whereas when I'm not, when there is something that is not right, either spiritually or emotionally, then I feel like I'm off centre, like I'm off on this side adjunct and just going nowhere.

Others used more concrete examples and invoked an almost endless list of criteria in talking about being balanced or centred. Some of these have been noted in the literature on alternative therapies. For instance, balanced/centred people lack stress (Coward 1989; Furnham and Bhagrath 1993); are loving and tolerant of themselves and others (McGuire and Kantor 1987); are moderate; have heightened mental alertness; are open; live in the present; and/or have an enhanced awareness of themselves and others. While some informants only referred to one or two of these requirements, most made use of several of them. Most popular was the belief that being balanced, and consequently healthy, means living without stress. For example, Betty pointed out that an imbalance in self caused by stress can manifest itself in physical problems:

> Ill health in a sense I would say starts on a level other than the physical and eventually manifests itself on the physical plane because of other things like, perhaps, the stress load on your emotions. Cancer [and] arthritis are two main diseases that are triggered eventually through certainly poor

diet over many years, pollutants and this sort of thing. Your chemicals: they play a big factor, but to me stress is just as big a factor, if not more so, than the rest of it.

Several informants linked the idea of developing heightened awareness of oneself and one's environment with the ability to avoid stress. According to Richard, "You're aware of yourself and you're moving through things in a clear, relaxed and fluid manner, and you're not spending your time, your gut isn't eating you away." Similarly, Randal told me, "You need to take time for M E spelling me. You need to slow down. Stop doing for everybody else. You've got to stop burning the candle at both ends. Your body is shutting down and saying take time for me, take time to slow down." And Lucy said this: "What I have to do is avoid a lot of stress because stress puts even more stress upon your health. So you have to become a lot more aware of your environment, a lot more aware of your own personal reactions, and if you do then you're fine."

For Betty, being healthy means not only avoiding stress but also being a tolerant, loving person towards yourself and others. She said: "To me health is just being as good and loving, sensible and forgiving, and caring and reasonable, person as you can with all things, and with all people, and most of all with yourself." Similarly, Lorraine believes that achieving the balance necessary to health entails being loving. She told me: "The trick in life is always to send out as much positive energy, the love energy, that we don't get our teeter-totter out of balance." Further, Hanna described how achieving balance through alternative health made her more moderate in her behaviour and emotional reactions as well as giving her tolerance, patience, and a heightened awareness of others. In her words,

I very rarely go up and down, I don't get over-excited about things. You learn not to question what's happening to you, being just a little bit more psychic, you have more ESP and you reach an awareness of people. And it's also a tolerance, [I'm] a lot more patient than I was before.

For a few of the people who took part in this research, being balanced, and consequently healthy, means living in the present or for the moment. According to Randal, "I've learned to celebrate life. I've learned to savour the moment, being in the present and taking care of myself."

Some of the people I spoke with extended the concept of balance beyond themselves to include what Lowenberg (1992:27) terms an "ecological view." In other words, their understanding of balance in the self includes balance between themselves and their personal environment (physical space, social structures, and personal relationships), the natural environment, and/or the universe. For example, Randal explained how he and his personal environment had become unbalanced: "I'd come down with walking pneumonia. I said: 'This is not worth it.' So I cleared myself of the roommate situation, I cleared myself of the job situation, and I started a cleansing." Other informants conceptualized balance in the self as something that incorporates balance with nature. According to Hanna, "Everything in life has a life force. In yoga it's called *prana*, in *tai chi* it's called *qi*[1] and *qi* means energy, that's all it is. I think every thing is a balance, nature is a balance, we should be in balance with nature." Finally, a few of the people who spoke with me saw balance in the self as something that necessitates balance with the universe. As was the case with healing energy, those informants who believe health to be dependent on a balance between the self and the universe are also more likely to espouse alternative spiritual beliefs. In Lorraine's words,

> Understanding the laws of the way that the universe works. I think of it as universal energy, and when we're cast out as souls for this learning experience, there's one tiny spark. It's still a part of fire even though it's separate from the fire. In other words, the teeter-totter always has to be in balance.

But how is balance in the body and balance in the self actualized? For most of these informants, the key to balance is control.

Control

For most of the people who took part in this research, achieving wholeness and balance, in short, means control. Control in turn means two things: taking control and being subject to self-control. Taking control of the healing process also includes having options and having the autonomy to make decisions, a belief found in other research on lay perspectives on alternative therapies (Sharma 1992). Finally, being subject to self-control means controlling one's thoughts, behaviours, and emotional reactions.

For almost all the people who participated in this study, alternative health means taking control of the healing process. For some of these people this means wresting control away from medical professionals. For instance, Nora told me, "Even when people want to take responsibility, often they're not allowed to because allopathic medicine really does have a lot to do with that." And Marie said this: "Take charge of [your] own wellness. Take an active role in your own healing and with mainstream medicine they take that away from you." Similarly, Simon related his experience of struggling with his doctors for control over his healing: "But the doctors, some didn't agree with chiropractic, some thought it was too harsh on the body. Some just had a general distrust of chiropractors and again they were trying to take the control out of my hands and putting it into their hands."

For other informants, taking control also means having options and making decisions. For example, Laura told me that alternative "health is the freedom to make the choices that I've made," and Lucy said this:

> If a doctor says: 'This is what's wrong, it's serious, it's chronic, it's life-threatening,' I may respect his education and his experience but he's not infallible. Therefore, why would I not go and have one or two more other estimates to say: 'Do you see this from the same perspective?' I mean, if I'm going to die, I'm going to die, that's my problem. It's the method in which I go from health to death that I want to have a choice in.

For still other informants, taking control means asking questions and getting second opinions. As Jane put it, "I think everybody needs to be a consumer and take responsibility for what they buy. You don't buy a pig in a poke and you don't buy a diagnosis without questioning it." Lorraine also stressed the value of taking control via questioning initial diagnoses:

> I think it's up to you, the individual, to get second opinions if, in your intu-itive part, your gut feeling, if it doesn't sit right. Like that D and C [Dilation and Curettage] didn't sit right. I went out and asked more opinions and then I made a decision that I was not having that D and C.

Montbriand and Laing (1991) argue that taking control of health and healing can also include the option of deciding to relinquish control to a practitioner. One informant, Laura, equated taking control with trusting her midwife enough to hand over control to her:

> I had so much trust and faith in her [the midwife] that during the delivery anything that she would have suggested I probably would have gone along with because I knew that what she would suggest would not be invasive

and would only be done if absolutely necessary. I felt like I was in control and had passed that control to her for that period of time.

Finally, for many of these informants, taking control of your health means doing your own research (Sharma 1992). According to Jenny, "If I'm going to an acupuncturist, I have to spend as long learning about all the meridians." Finally, Raymond connected the ability to make decisions with doing your own research and being well informed about your health problem:

> Read up on it, educate yourself, make your own decisions. Do this for you. You've got to take control, know what you're putting in your body, know the side effects. Is it worth the quality of life loss for quantity? It's a difficult toss-up and it's a decision.

The literature shows that people feel that the alternative model of health allows them to take control (Furnham and Forey 1994; Kelner and Wellman 1997; Kronenfeld and Wasner 1982; Vincent and Furnham 1996; Pawluch et al. 1994; Sharma 1992). However, what is less conspicuous in the literature, and quite blatant throughout these interviews, is that taking control of your health in practice means engaging in a great deal of self-control (Coward 1989; Kelner and Wellman 1997; Pawluch et al. 1994). Furthermore, while taking control of your health may mean having choices as to how your health is cared for, it also means assuming total responsibility for your health status (Deierlein 1994; Lowenberg 1992; Pawluch et al. 1998a). For instance, Brenda had this to say: "I think I have to make the effort. Maybe alternative [health] is everybody's responsibility and they have to do it themselves." And Lindsay said this: "There's not enough people who are willing to make the commitment of their own health care. And I really believe that people are responsible for their own health and you have to say: 'Well this isn't working' or 'What else is there?' or 'I did some reading on this.'" Lucy also emphasized that under this alternative model, health is a matter of what individuals are willing to do for themselves: "You're aware when things are not in balance and once you know you have to make a decision: Do I want it to stay in balance, or to get worse, or am I prepared to go back and correct it?"

In practical terms, what taking control of, or responsibility for, your health means for these people is a great deal of self-monitoring and self-control, controlling everything from lifestyles to attitudes.[2] For example, controlling stress is an important component of such an alternative model of health (Coward 1989; Furnham and Bhagrath 1993). According to Jane, "I analysed these ulcers. What causes ulcers but stress? Because it's not my diet. So it was just a matter of sitting back and saying, 'Hold it, I'll do my best at school. If I get an A wonderful, if I don't so what?'"

In addition, taking control of your healing means making lifestyle changes (Furnham and Kirkcaldy 1996; Yates et al. 1993). For many of these informants this means controlling their diet and changing the way they eat and drink. As Marie put it, "If somebody's drinking thirty cups of coffee a day and they're having trouble sleeping and they can't relax, well maybe look at your lifestyle." Similarly, Laura told me how she monitors what she eats: "I'm not a vegetarian, but if I have the choice between white rice and brown rice, I'll eat brown. There are very few processed foods in our house." Finally, Hanna talked about eliminating what she defines as unhealthy food from her diet: "Diet is my number one thing. What you put into your body is what affects yourself. I'm very strict on taking fats out of the system, sodium, sugars." Controlling the way they eat and drink also entails controlling the way they shop for food. For instance, Pam said, "I used to read labels to begin with; I read them now even more. You have to learn all the other little names that mean the same thing for the same foods."

For other informants self-control has more to do with controlling smoking, drinking, and other conduct they now perceive as bad habits. For instance, Marie, Greg, and Randal all told me of behaviours they engaged in that they now see as unhealthy under their alternative model of health. According to Marie, "I still smoke. I used to smoke a pack, a pack and a half a day; I smoke maybe six or seven cigarettes a day now. I used to be a very heavy drinker. I gave that up." Similarly, Greg told me,

> I was able to try some acupuncture and I have to admit I did notice a fair improvement. It wasn't a permanent improvement, but that probably means that there is still something goofy with the body. I'm just going along following all the bad habits I may have picked up along the way.

For Randal also, alternative health requires control of "bad habits":

> If you're going to be out in the cold bundle up! Common sense stuff, you know? Take care of yourself! Eat properly; eat the whole thing! And I was

partying too much at that time. I was studying, I was partying, I was pushing myself. It was a slap on the hand to say 'Slow down.'

Moreover, if individuals' lifestyles are not making them sick, their mind or emotional reactions may likely do so. Therefore, alternative health requires control over one's "mind, attitudes, and belief systems" (Lowenberg 1992:25). According to Richard, "You change destructive behaviour [and] destructive beliefs" in order to pursue alternative health. For just as the mind has the ability to heal the person, under this alternative model, it can also make one sick (McGuire 1987; McGuire and Kantor 1987). For instance, Trudy said, "I realized that there was a lot more to it in terms of the whole psychology. I could understand that my body was responding to my own thinking." And Lorraine told me,

> Whether cancer cells or different types of cells, it's the stress and negativity that sets these things in motion. Sure they could be in five hundred people; maybe four hundred of them will set them in motion. The other one hundred realize that the thinking process keeps those last one hundred from setting their cells in motion. What happens with negative thinking is that you end up with problems. It becomes your heart problems; rigid thinking becomes your arthritis. Each of these thinking patterns creates a different disease in the body.

Similarly, Betty highlighted the causal role in ill health played by negative thought patterns:

> To me any negative emotions or feelings are a garden for seeds of ill health that you're planting, and somewhere, whether it's ten years down the line, it's going to catch up with you as those negative seeds grow into bigger and bigger negative plants.

Finally, for some of the people who spoke with me, *healthy* self-control means controlling their emotional reactions. Brenda, for instance, stated the following:

> I started a lot of exploring with different therapies, changing my lifestyle. I was always expecting other people to change. I would always react to situations. I realized that I was in control and only I could change the way I responded to situations.

THE IMPLICATIONS OF ALTERNATIVE HEALTH BELIEFS

For the people who participated in this research, health and healing are an ongoing, concomitant process. Their alternative model of health is made up of three fundamental conceptual categories: holism, balance, and control. To be healthy under this model means that one experiences and exhibits unity of, as well as balance between, mind, body, and spirit. The category of balance also includes the notions of unity with, and balance between, the self and others, the self and nature, and/or the self and the universe. What being balanced comes down to is taking control of one's health and healing, which in turn means being subject to considerable self-control. This model of health is one for which the people who spoke with me have nothing but praise, in contrast to their negative appraisals of allopathic medicine. Throughout the interviews they conveyed to me their belief that participation in alternative therapies has improved not only their health but also their lives. My intent here is not to question the validity of their beliefs in this regard, but rather to submit the components of this alternative model of health to critical analysis. In doing so, what becomes clear is that there are other, less positive, implications for the individual of an adoption of such an ideology of health.

Research has shown that part of what lay people value about alternative therapies is that they are based on an ideology where health is understood as comprising more than just human biology (Furnham and Smith 1988; Pawluch et al.1994; Schneirov and Geczik 1996). Likewise, amongst the positive aspects attributed to these informants' alternative model of health is its emphasis on a holistic understanding of health and healing. A holistic approach to health care is something that the informants desire and something they feel is woefully lacking in allopathic medicine. However, for the individual who adopts such an alternative model of health, holism has its price. For example, one implication for the individual of the pursuit of this form of holistic health is that participation in alternative therapies can be, as McGuire (1988) points out, incredibly labour intensive. To illustrate, Pam's daughter was diagnosed by their naturopath as having several allergies and sensitivities, many of them to food. In the following account, Pam describes the resources she invests in providing an environment that she believes is healthy for her daughter:

> I knew that she had a lactose problem. We also knew that she didn't like eggs,
> so we had eliminated them out of her diet. So I said to [the naturopath]: 'OK,

fluoride?' He said: 'Basically, you don't drink the town water now.' So I truck to [another town] and bring my water in. I had to go and find toothpaste that doesn't have fluoride in it. She's linked to what they call the five major North American foods: corn, wheat, eggs, yeast, milk. She also reacts to chicken. I make turkey for her when we have chicken at home. I'm at the point of getting a rooster and trying rooster because from the reading that I've done, they say that some people can eat capon, and rooster capons are very hard to come by. She doesn't like soy bean and I sort of panicked—what do I feed this child? I have the luxury of being at home with my kids so I can spend that extra time making sure that there's baking and the menu planning. I don't know how a person who works full-time could manage all of this because it's very labour intensive.

Here Pam reflects on the time and effort she expends in pursuit of alternative health for her daughter, but what is also implicit is that time and effort are not the only resources involved in seeking alternative health; Pam also invests a great deal of money, in terms of the cost of specialty foods, transportation, and the cost of privately obtained naturopathic treatment. Clearly, a problematic aspect of this model of alternative health for the individual is the sheer amount of labour and expense it entails. Consequently, alternative health is restricted to those with the resources available to pursue it.

In addition, a key aspect of holism that can have negative consequences for the individual is the notion of balance, as it is defined by the people I spoke with. For example, just as the World Health Organization's definition of health[3] has been criticized for being impossible to achieve, so too is holistic health when it rests upon a concept of balance entailing a never-ending list of criteria. Therefore, a negative implication for the individual is the potential for frustration and unwarranted feelings of failure when he or she is unable to attain balance. It is questionable whether conceiving of health as the process of healing provides sufficient protection for individuals from the potential harmful impact of the unrealistic expectations for health implicit in a concept of balance that is forever beyond their ability to attain.

Another feature of alternative models of health, which people who use these types of therapies find beneficial, is that they are said to provide individuals with the opportunity to take control of their own healing process (Kelner and Wellman 1997; Vincent and Furnham 1996; Sharma 1990, 1992). Consistent with these findings, most informants said that taking control of their health and healing is something they desire and an option they feel is not possible within allopathic approaches to health care. However, for these people, taking control, in essence, means self-control, and therein lies the potential for self-blame for failure to eliminate what they now define as unhealthy conduct (Furnham and Kirkcaldy 1996; Glik 1988). For example, several informants admitted feeling guilty when they are unable to purge certain behaviours from their lifestyles. In Lorraine's words,

> I'm feeling guilty when I mix the starch and the meat together, when I have that bag of chips that I hide from the rest of the world and sneak when nobody else is around. *I know I'm being bad*, but I'm not as bad as I used to be. I used to have chips every night, now I might have them once a week. Hopefully I can even eradicate that in time. (emphasis mine)

Other informants also felt guilty when they failed to follow their alternative healing regimes. For instance, when I asked Richard if he meditated, he told me, "I do and I don't do it as much as *I should*"; and Lindsay said, "I'm supposed to be taking, *I'm not very good* about doing this, but I'm supposed to be taking some fish oil right now" (emphases mine). Therefore, and in contrast to these people's beliefs about the benign nature of alternative healing, this alternative model of health has considerable potential to produce "iatrogenic" effects in the form of guilt, self-blame, and other types of emotional distress (Illich 1975:22).

Furthermore, implicit in the concept of taking control is the assumption that individuals take full responsibility for the state of their health (Coward 1989; McGuire and Kantor 1987; Sharma 1992). Assigning total responsibility to the individual makes such an alternative ideology of health vulnerable to criticism usually associated with the biomedical model of health. While Gillet (1994) asserts that the alternative model is less punitive than the biomedical model, several other authors conclude that both models are equally reductionist where responsibility for sickness is concerned (Berliner and Salmon 1979a, 1979b; Coward 1989; Sharma 1992). In other words, both the biomedical and alternative models blame the victim of ill health through location of the sources and solutions to health problems solely within the individual. For example, McGuire and Kantor (1987:236) describe an episode where a woman who participated in their research explained how she was being taught by her healing circle to accept her paralysis as her chosen path.

Moreover, in individualizing health problems, this alternative model of health turns attention away from the social factors that produce illness and disease (Sharma 1992). In one sense, such an alternative ideology of health is even less attentive to the social production of illness than is the biomedical model. For instance, epidemiologists, at least, recognize a relationship between the environment and disease, whereas under this alternative model, it is not the environment, but rather how one reacts to one's environment, that is the cause of ill health. Nowhere are these forms of reductionism more apparent than in this alternative ideology's identification of thought patterns as the aetiological starting point for illness and disease. For example, Randal told me, "We have to correct our thinking. I wasn't positive at all. There's a psychological background to each of these diseases; diabetics, some of them are very similar people, so they become sour people. With arthritis some of them are very bitter." Such a belief in locating the genesis of health problems within the individual's mind is as reductionist as the biomedical model of health's emphasis on explaining ill health through individual physiology (Coward 1989; McGuire 1987).

Finally, in contrast, and in addition to health benefits, espousing such an alternative model of health can have positive consequences for the individual's subjective perceptions of self. For instance, self and identity may be positively affected through adoption of this alternative model of health when the ideology contained within it is used as a mechanism for constructing a healthy sense of self.

NOTES

1. Pronounced "chi."
2. See Crawford (1984) for the wider cultural implications of the belief that health is achieved through self-control.
3. "A state of complete physical, mental, and social well-being and not merely the absence of disease or infirmity" (Armstrong and Armstrong 1996:13–14).

CHAPTER SIX

Alternative Healing and the Self

In participation in alternative health care, as well as through interaction with alternative practitioners and other lay users of these therapies, the people who took part in this research began to adopt alternative ideologies of health and healing—ideologies that can have, at times, profound implications for individuals' subjective perceptions of self. For instance, Schneirov and Geczik (1996:638) write that the networks of alternative therapy use that these people develop are a "significant source of new meanings and identities." Similarly, Pawluch et al. (1994:71) write that for some of their informants,

> the benefits of using alternative therapies went beyond improved health. Participation in therapies that emphasized holistic health often served as a catalyst for broader personal transformation: changes in identity ... that extended beyond specific health issues.

Similarly, the ideologies contained within the models of health and healing espoused by the people who spoke with me impacted on them in two particular ways. Some became so enamoured of alternative approaches to health care that they sought training in these therapies, beginning the process of taking on the identity of alternative practitioners or healers. Others experienced changes in perceptions of self as a result of their participation in alternative therapies. For many of these informants, the ideology contained within their alternative models of health and healing became a mechanism through which they were able to construct a healthy sense of self.

ADOPTING A HEALER IDENTITY

One type of change in identity experienced by the people I spoke with is that which is engendered through the process of adoption of a healer identity,[1] a process noted in other research on lay use of alternative therapies (Sharma 1992). Becoming a healer has implications for identity as, in Becker's (1970a:293) words, changing one's profession entails that the individual undergo adult socialization, which in turn "can be ... conceptualized as a matter of change to self." For over half of the people who took part in this study, participation in alternative therapies led them to begin the process of becoming an alternative practitioner or healer. This process can be conceptualized as a continuum of identity change that spans taking courses in order to self-treat through to formal training to become a certified practitioner (see Figure 6.1).

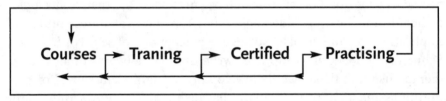

Figure 6.1. The Healer Continuum

The arrow that connects the end of the continuum to its beginning in Figure 6.1 is intended to show that once certified and practising, alternative healers often take new courses in order to practice additional therapies. The downward arrows denote that beginning the process of becoming an alternative practitioner does not mean that one will necessarily follow it through to the end. Rather, people may pause or stop at any point along this continuum of identity change. For example, some of the informants sought out alternative healing courses for therapeutic purposes only and had no plans to engage in formal, certified training. In Jane's words, "I've taken *reiki* courses and things like that so [my husband has] seen me laying on the living room carpet with my crystals and my healing stones out and doing my own thing." Likewise, almost all of the informants who identified themselves as alternative practitioners began the process of adopting this identity by initially taking courses in alternative therapies in order to address their own health problems. Take the case of Lorraine:

I have taken the *reiki* and now I have my first and second levels.... There's another place you can go. I'm going there in August and they offer all kinds of self-awareness courses. I go down there for positive thinking courses, health courses. The one I went to was healing, channelling, and meditation.

If the individual continues along this continuum, the next stage he or she reaches is formal training in one or other alternative therapies. For example, Lucy was in training to become a reflexologist and told me she hoped to practice this therapy professionally:

I'm now taking my courses for reflexology. I would like to practice the reflexology definitely and maybe *shiatsu* massage. I've never tried that but I've heard so many people comment on how well it made them feel. But with reflexology, if I could help somebody feel as good as it made me feel. I think what it does is it helps the individual to become in touch with themselves and allows the body to repair itself.

While training in a therapy can lead to certification, not all informants who complete training in a particular therapy intend to practice it. For instance, Jenny underwent training to become a certified hypnotherapist but had no intention of practising professionally. The important point however, is that it was her belief in these therapies that brought her this far along the continuum. According to Jenny,

Someone recommended hypnotherapy for something that was on my mind. I was complaining and this person started talking about it and so I decided to go and see about it and *I was so completely taken with the process* that I eventually ended up taking a course in certified clinical hypnotherapy and in neurolinguistics programming. (emphasis mine)

The degree of formality involved in the training and certification processes taken up by these people varied. Some practised therapies that were certified or regulated to some degree. For instance, Hanna explained her own experience to me:

I'm a yoga therapist and a reflexologist. I went to college. The brochures were offering a yoga course that was on four different levels and it took eighteen months to complete. In the course I also got taught a little

reflexology so that kind of stayed on the back burner until I got everything
working with the yoga. And after I did that I decided to look for a course there.
I went for my reflexology, which was a six months course, a certified course.

Similarly, after using the Feldenkrais method informally, Roger described how
he sought formal training: "So I was using it also with handicapped people,
just in a very informal way, and then I decided to get trained in it and did the
second North American training that existed." Other informants trained and
practised without formal certification or regulation of any type. For example,
Natalie told me that she practised alternative healing independently out of her
home: "I would try to heal people with my mind from a distance, or with my
hands from a distance, and I was finding it was working."

In addition to inspiring these people to take courses in alternative therapies,
and to become certified as alternative practitioners, deepening commitment
to alternative ideologies of health and healing also motivated several informants to make the decision to practice alternative health care professionally. For
these people, a key encounter with an alternative practitioner reinforced their
commitment to these therapies (Deierlein 1994). For example, Scott and
Natalie told me about meetings with alternative practitioners that launched
them on the road to becoming healers themselves. According to Scott,

> I met this woman who was a practitioner. She was really inspiring, she was
> amazing, she was full of life and joy and she had her own health and she
> had her practice room and she had her own world and she travelled all over
> the world and did this and that and met all these amazing healers, and I
> had never really thought about healing up until this time. But I realized
> as I was getting to know this woman, it was like: 'Oh my god! I want to
> become a healer.'

Similarly, Natalie told me,

> I went to a healer when I first moved up here and he told me I was a
> healer, and of course I just laughed because I really didn't know what a
> healer was. He's sensational, he was really good. We just sat there for fif-
> teen minutes and we talked. We talked about nutrition and everything else
> and then he said, 'Natalie, you're a healer.'

These informants also saw particular therapeutic experiences as turning points that motivated them to become practitioners in their own right. For instance, after experiencing successful acupuncture treatments, Simon made the decision to leave medical school and train to become an acupuncturist:

> I was on every kind of muscle relaxant, painkiller, sleep aid, everything. Nothing was working. I was taking them by the handfuls. My chiropractor also does acupuncture so we tried acupuncture and within two weeks I was off all the medications and I said: 'You know, I'm going into this field' and that's what I did. Said goodbye to formal education and mainstream medicine and went into the alternative.

These key encounters and experiences are important because it is through them that alternative ideology is more deeply internalized by the individual. In other words, an individual's "commitment to a healer/client relationship," in particular, is instrumental in the adoption of alternative belief systems (Deierlein 1994:180). Deepening commitment to alternative ideology is, in turn, what propels people along the continuum of identity change. For example, it was the intensity of Marie's belief in alternative therapies that inspired her to become an alternative practitioner: "I became a certified reflexologist because *I believe in those things so much*" (emphasis mine).

CHANGES IN SELF-PERCEPTION

Adopting a healer identity was one type of self-change experienced by the people who took part in this study; however, it was not the only one. For many informants, participation in alternative therapies, and adoption of alternative health and healing ideologies, led to changes in their subjective perceptions of self. In particular, it allowed them to re-define aspects of personal identity, that "unique collection of life history items that comes to be attached to the individual" (Goffman 1963:57). That participation in alternative approaches to health care can have this effect has been observed in other research on the users of alternative therapies (Csordas 1983; Easthope 1993; Glik 1988 1990; McGuire 1983, 1987; Pawluch et al.1994). For instance, in describing the use of creative visualization among participants in a metaphysical healing group (MHG), Glik (1988:1201) reports that "In MHGs images of light emanating from and surrounding the self protected from dark forces and to some degree *transformed self* and others" (emphasis mine).

In a similar vein, several of the people who participated in this research perceived changes to themselves as a result of their experiences with alternative therapies. According to Natalie, "I heard about that [course] through the healing circle; somebody mentioned to me that they were going to take it. The three in our group went and we've all completely changed." Betty also experienced change in herself through participation in alternative approaches to health and healing: "That was a lot of years ago and I was barely getting started. I'm sure a different person now than to what I was." While several of these people told me they had experienced change to self through their use of alternative health care, there were variations in the degree to which different informants felt that participation in these therapies had affected them. Some told me that using alternative therapies altered their entire lives or their whole selves. Others perceived these changes to self to have occurred primarily on the level of their value systems or their personalities.

For instance, some informants felt that using alternative approaches to health and healing impacted on their lives in some fundamental and pervasive way. Witness Grace: "I can only speak for myself but it has changed my life. It has changed my life." Consistent with the tenets of the alternative model of health and healing, these people saw this change as embracing all levels of the person: mind, body, and spirit. In Hanna's words,

> The idea is that since you're affecting the whole nervous system and hence the whole body you can have profound physical and emotional change happening. If I have a holistic perspective I know that I'm also working with someone's emotions and their whole self.... It's not like you're just doing a physical thing: you change them emotionally and you change their attitude.

Natalie also told me that her alternative therapies are oriented towards healing a person's whole life: "Their life, mentally and physically and spiritually." She went on to describe the changes to self she and her companions experienced through participation in alternative health care: "We've all completely changed, physically we've changed, we look different, younger, we've got more vitality, more energy, we feel alive." As the interviews progressed it became clear that for many it was not the circumstances of their lives that had changed, but that they believed that their entire selves could be, or had been, transformed. For example, Roger told me the following:

I quickly saw that it had applications for the work I was doing with the handicapped people, just for working on the general organization of the nervous system, the musculature, *the organization of the person in general. Personality,* all that type of thing.... One of the reasons I think that the Feldenkrais work touched me so personally when I experienced the work were some of the effects on just balancing and organizing the system, the nervous system, *the person.* (emphases mine)

For most informants, however, the changes to self they perceived related to different aspects of their personal identities; specifically, changes to value systems and personalities.

Changes in Personality

Almost all of the people who spoke with me felt that their use of alternative therapies resulted in changes to one or more aspects of their personalities. For instance, Laura felt she had gained confidence and become a more assertive person through her use of alternative therapies: "At the time I wasn't a very assertive person, I don't believe that any more about myself.... I have a lot more confidence in myself now." While Laura's perception of change to her personality was relatively circumscribed, most other informants experienced this change as more or less all-encompassing. For example, Pam believed that an alternative approach resulted in what she saw as a remarkable change in her daughter's entire personality:

I removed all the wheat that you could just see, the bread, the buns. I hadn't really removed that hidden wheat that's in everything. And within three weeks there was a remarkable change, change in personality, the temper tantrums left, the disorganization left. She was never a morning person, now she's up at quarter to seven.

Hanna also believed that several aspects of her personality had changed and that she had become a calmer, more tolerant, more contented, and a less worried person:

I'm a lot more level. When you do yoga for several years you go through different levels of experiences and you learn not to question what's happening to you.... It means more contentment because you're not worried. I feel a lot more self-sufficient, I don't worry about the future any more.

Similarly, Brenda believed she had become a more patient and tolerant person, less argumentative and judgmental, more honest with herself, and, in general, happier:

I don't judge anybody; the other thing is happiness. I was totally miserable, that's totally changed. Also relationships, I was always angry with something, I was never satisfied, everything was wrong. Our lives were just bitching and complaining at each other and now we don't ever. I'm very patient, I'm not in the least bit stressful. I used to plan a lot, I used to worry a lot. And I'm really honest now; I never used to be honest with myself.

The changes Betty saw in her personality included becoming more confident and calmer, as well as less fearful and worried. She told me, "Things don't bother me nearly as deeply or the same as they would have. I'm a lot calmer, happier, healthier. I have a confidence in myself, in my ability, in my life, that I didn't used to have. I've got no fears." Some of the informants who espouse non-mainstream religious beliefs felt that participation in alternative health care led to them becoming more intuitive. For instance, Hanna said that one of the changes she experienced in her personality was "being just a little bit more psychic. You have more ESP and you reach an awareness of people." Similarly, Brenda said,

I think it's intuition ... I think once you become spiritually aware or are beyond the two dimensions of body and mind I think you can, ... it surprises me because I never used to be very intuitive. I even said to her [alternative practitioner], 'How will I know when I'm intuitive? I'll never be intuitive.' She said, 'It will come'—and it has.

Finally, Jenny pointed out that it was the changes to personality she experienced as a result of her use of alternative therapies that led to physical benefits for her. She said: "It's given me at certain times a greater composure, ability to survive, openness to others and just a greater sense of well-being which goes through to the way I feel physically."

Changes in Value Systems

Some informants felt that their use of alternative therapies resulted in a realignment of their priorities or value systems. Those who perceived their values to have changed were more likely to espouse non-mainstream religious beliefs. For example, both Hanna, who is a Buddhist, and Lorraine, who follows new age spirituality, felt they had changed in terms of the value they placed on material things. For instance, Hanna said: "It's a completely different way of thinking. Material things take less and less emphasis. I feel as if I've wasted so much time on things that weren't important." Likewise, Lorraine told me: "I also have to be able to say that it's only material things and walk away. The lives that I care for are more important than what's in their hand. There was a point in my life that I could have never said that, they're only things, they do not matter." The important point, however, is that given the relationship these informants see between their spirituality and their use of alternative therapies, these changes to their value systems have as much to do with alternative ideologies of health and healing as they do with non-mainstream spiritual beliefs.

Whether the changes these people perceive occur on the level of value systems, personality, or in the whole person, they are experienced as positive change. In short, the informants are becoming better people. According to Lindsay,

> I got my orthotics and balanced my feet and started having my chiropractic done and balanced my hips. I think it's important for everybody to find things that help them *be the best person they can*. That's why I'm exploring it [alternative therapies], cause I want to be the *best possible person I can*. (emphases mine)

Similarly, Natalie said, "They're like different human beings, they're just different, *much better human beings,*" and Richard told me alternative healing is "the ability to see the change in other people's mental physical and spiritual state and making them ... aware ... *they're better* because of it" (emphases mine). Again, it is the ideology contained within their alternative models of health and healing that makes them better people. In Hanna's words,

> Yoga philosophy is to be basically a very good person with high moral standards. Love your neighbour as yourself, that type of thing, but a lot

more self-discipline, mental and physical discipline, and to be a nice person, treat other people the best way you can, don't judge people, and *I suppose the philosophy is to improve yourself.* (emphasis mine)

Moreover, in addition to helping them be better people, the ideology contained within these informants' alternative models of health and healing can become a mechanism for healing the self.

HEALING THE SELF

McGuire (1987:376) contends that "the very rhetorics of healing in modern Western societies emphasize individual choice and transformation." In particular, alternative approaches to healing have been observed to have this type of self-transformative potential (Glik 1988,1990; McGuire 1983; Pawluch et al. 1994; Stambolovic 1996; Ullman 1979). For instance, Easthope (1993:294) asserts that "The healer's task is to reconstruct ... individuals in a mode that provides them with the ability to manage their disease." However, O'Connor (1995:28) points out that "physical recovery may not be the most important outcome" of alternative healing. Consequently, the reconstruction of the individual engendered through his or her participation in alternative therapies does not merely enable the person to better cope with disease, but can also provide the individual with the means to change his or her self-perceptions. Moreover, for the people I spoke with, self-healing not only means developing the ability to relieve one's own physical, emotional, or spiritual ailments; it also means acquiring the ability to heal the self. In particular, they are reshaping their personal identity, that which is unique to the individual (Goffman 1963). They are recasting their perceptions of self to account for perceived changes in identity from sick to healthy and from negative to positive. They are engaged in what Corbin and Strauss (1987:264) call biographical work, which includes "its review, maintenance, repair and alteration," where alteration refers to "transitions to identity which are prescribed or at least permitted within the persons' established universe of discourse" (Berger 1963, Travisano 1981:244); this is in contrast to notions of conversions which imply that one's past identity is completely jettisoned in favour of a new identity (Berger 1963; Travisano 1981). Thus these people have constructed a new sense of self which they incorporate within the totality of their personal identities.

McGuire (1987:374) contends that the symbolic embodiment of ideology has the power to change people. She asserts that "through rituals and symbols of transformation, believers experience changes in themselves," and Glik (1990:160) likewise concludes that it is through "the adoption of strong ... *beliefs* [that] individual dramas of change, real or imagined, are realized" (emphasis mine).[2] Similarly, Csordas (1983:346,356) argues that "meaningful and convincing discourse brings about a transformation of the phenomenological conditions under which the patient exists and experiences suffering and distress. This movement amounts to a reconstruction of self." And for many of the people who took part in this research, it is the ideology underpinning their alternative models of health and healing that serves as a mechanism for constructing healthy self-perceptions, or what Lindsey (1996:466) calls "health within illness."[3]

To illustrate, a fundamental assumption of these informant's alternative health and healing ideologies, which has implications for transformations of self, is the belief that to be healthy is to be engaged in the process of healing. Accordingly, for these people, being in a state of health does not depend exclusively on physical soundness as defined under biomedicine. Rather, under their alternative models of health and healing, "to be healed is not necessarily the same as to be cured" (McGuire and Kantor 1987:233). For instance, Jane told me, "Health to me is not necessarily a physical definition of health but just a sense of your own well-being." And Betty said that alternative health is

> A beautiful state of well-being on every level of your being, the physical level, your emotional level, your medical level, your spiritual level. And they're all completely part of you, and all completely intertwined, and you can't really be healthy on one level if you're not on the others. But by no means just the physical level because actually ill health starts on a level other than the physical and eventually manifests on the physical.

Thus, under their alternative ideologies of health and healing, "the disease is rendered secondary" (Coward 1989:47). In contrast, biomedicine defines ill health as "a deviation from normal biological functioning" (Mishler 1989:3) that greatly reduces the boundaries within which one can be healthy. Moreover, an attendant consequence of biomedically defined ill health is the loss of self engendered by disease, chronic illness, and disability (Bury 1982, 1991; Charmaz 1983, 1991; Corbin and Strauss 1988).

Under these informants' alternative model of health, perceiving oneself as healthy becomes an achievable reality, as compared to the more limited prognoses for self available under biomedicine, as it provides the ideological means of repairing or reconstructing the lost or damaged self.

More precisely, it is the assumption that alternative health is manifested in engagement in an ongoing process of healing which allows one to be healthy even in the face of disease or infirmity. For instance, Grace saw herself as healthy despite the fact that she is paralysed. A further reflection of their belief that to be healthy is to be continually engaged in healing is that the changes to self these people perceive are experienced as a dynamic, rather than static, process. According to Betty, "I'm still changing, very much so. I'm much better within myself than I was even a year ago." Natalie also understood the changes to self she perceived as an ongoing process: "It should be permanent *as long as we keep healing*" (emphasis mine). While this core assumption is what ultimately allows the people who participated in this research to perceive themselves as healthy despite the presence of biomedically defined ill health, different informants emphasized different elements of their alternative models of health and healing as the particular ideological mechanisms they employed for this type of change to self. For example, Laura is able to see herself as healthy by invoking the alternative healing notion of the body's ability to heal itself: "I'm healthy right now despite the fact that I have a cold because I know that my body is strong enough to fight it." In contrast, Randal has a strong sense of personal health, despite living with HIV, through his emphasis on holism, one component of these informants' alternative model of health. In his words, "It's mind, body, spirit, emotionally connecting it all. I'm doing that. I'm keeping that glow of health around me all the time."

This type of change to self is different from Charmaz's (1987:287) concept of the salvaged self, where "ill persons attempt to define self as positive and worthwhile, despite their reduced ability to function.... By this time they hold little hope of realizing typical adult identities in the outer world." It is different because the people who took part in this study have not given up hope of healthy selves because the ideology contained within their alternative models of health and healing gives them that hope. For example, in telling me about how a friend of his had reconstructed herself through participation in alternative therapies, Greg said,

> I know of case histories and *people who actually have rebuilt themselves.* She's functioning and confident now. Rebuilt is the best word I can think

of and he [the alternative practitioner] did it without making her take pills, without marginalizing her. Because if it's not treatable the doctors will say, 'Well, you're going to have to settle for this.' At least she had some hope and she had good reason for hope. (emphasis mine)

While many authors agree that a persistent appeal of alternative approaches to health and healing is that they offer people hope (Northcott 1994), there is debate as to just what the nature of this hope is. For instance, Kottow (1992) and Feigen and Tiver (1986) argue that alternative health care is dangerous because it gives people the false hope of curing what ails them. Conversely, others argue that alternative therapies offer people renewed hope that they will find a solution to their health problem (Murray and Rubel 1992). The relevant issue for these informants, however, is not whether or not their alternative models of health and healing provide them with valid or false hopes of a cure. Rather, it is that they offer the hope of constructing a healthy sense of self. Therefore, the hope held out by alternative approaches to health care comes in two forms: the hope of "different possibilities for alleviating human suffering" (Stambolovic 1996:603) certainly; but more importantly, from a symbolic interactionist perspective on the self, it is the hope of "changing psycho-social structures," among which is what we may consider to be a well role (Glik and Kronenfeld 1989). The hope of achieving healthy self-perceptions is possible for these people because unlike Charmaz's (1987:287) informants who were seeking a restored self, trying to "reconstruct ... the same *sense* of self they possessed before illness" (emphasis hers), these people sought to trans-form themselves, creating a new sense of self which they perceive as healthy.

The people who participated in this research experienced two types of identity change through their use of alternative therapies. For some, experiencing alternative approaches to health and health care led them to begin the process of taking on an alternative practitioner or healer identity. For others, participation in alternative health care resulted in changes to perceptions of self. What is central to both types of identity-change experienced by the people who spoke with me is the ideology contained within the alternative model of health and healing. This ideology is both the motivator for taking on the identity of an alternative healer and the mechanism through which they construct a healthy sense of self.

Notwithstanding the fact that these informants experienced positive changes to self through adoption of alternative ideologies of health and healing, participation in these forms of health care can also have a negative impact on identity. More precisely, a consequence of participation in alternative therapies is that people are often stigmatized for their use of what have been labelled "deviant systems of medicine" (Saks 1995:119). Therefore, while using alternative therapies can allow the individual to change their self-perceptions and transform their identities for the better, these benefits to self can come at the price of acquiring a deviant identity.

NOTES

1. My intent here is not an in-depth examination of the components of the alternative healer identity. Rather, I am concerned with what motivates these informants to begin, continue, or complete the process of adopting a healer identity. Interested readers should see Boon (1998); Cant and Calnan (1991); and Lowenberg (1992) for analyses of alternative practitioner identity.

2. Glik's (1990) characterization of the changes to self experienced by her informants as imagined is problematic. As Thomas and Thomas (1970:154) made plain, "If [people] define situations as real they are real in their consequences." Thus, for the people who participated in this study, the changes to self that they perceive are real in their experience.

3. While Lindsey (1996:466) does not identify the source of the beliefs that allowed her informants to find "health within illness" as alternative healing ideology, much of the data she presents in illustrating how her informants describe health are analogous to many of the components which make up the alternative model of health espoused by the people who spoke with me. For example, one woman who took part in her research defined health as "being in control of myself and making my own decisions" (Lindsey 1996:468).

CHAPTER SEVEN

Using Alternative Therapies: A Deviant Identity

The use of alternative therapies as deviant behaviour is neglected as an area of research, despite the fact that people who use so-called unorthodox therapies have consistently been ridiculed (Johnson 1999; Leech 1999; Miller et al. 1998; Moenkhoft et al. 1999), and their pursuit of these therapies described as "irrational [or] deviant illness behaviour" (Cassee 1970:389–91) by researchers, medical professionals, and others. For example, Hare (1993:40) equates a patient's disclosure of her use of acupuncture to her doctor with the Catholic confessional, and the use of alternative therapies with a sin that must be absolved: "She is confessing to her physician who absolves her, even confessing his own foray into the domain of the 'other.'" Further, Furnham and Smith (1988:689; Furnham and Beard 1995) suggest that the people they studied who visited homeopaths displayed more neuroses than those visiting a general practitioner, leading them to speculate that people who use alternative therapies may be members of a population of people who are "perpetually disturbed."

Despite the evidence that people who use alternative therapies continue to be labelled deviant, we still know little about how these people cope with the stigma conferred through use of these forms of health care. My focus here is on the means used by informants to reduce the stigma associated with their participation in alternative approaches to health and healing. In addition to describing the use of perennial methods of coping with stigma, such as managing disclosure and using humour (Davis 1961; Goffman 1963), I analyse informants' use of *accounts* as a technique of stigma management (Scott and Lyman 1981). In particular, I reflect on their use of retrospective reinterpretation of biography employed in their accounts of their participation in alternative therapies.

BIOGRAPHIES, ACCOUNTS AND RETROSPECTIVE REINTERPRETATION

In analysing how the people who took part in this research manage the stigma associated with participation in alternative therapies, I make use of concepts central to a symbolic interactionist understanding of self-identity; including Goffman's (1963) notion of personal identity, which includes "the individual's self-definitions forming his or her biography" (Charmaz 1987:284). One's self-defined biography is neither static nor fixed; rather, as Goffman (1963:62) points out, a salient feature of biographies is that they "are very subject to retrospective construction." Likewise, Berger (1963:56) writes that "We ourselves go on interpreting and reinterpreting our own life.... As we remember the past, we reconstruct it in accordance with our present ideas of what is important and what is not." This type of biographical work necessarily entails the use of accounts. In Scott and Lyman's (1981:357) words: "Every account is a manifestation of the under-lying negotiation of identities," and is no less so in negotiating deviant identities (emphasis theirs). According to Scott and Lyman (1981:343–344), "An account is a linguistic device employed whenever an action is subjected to valuative inquiry.... A statement made by a social actor to explain unanticipated or untoward behavior." There are two general categories of accounts: excuses and justifications. These categories differ in that justifications are accounts in which the actor "accepts responsibility for the act ... but denies the pejorative quality associated with it ... [while] excuses are socially approved vocabularies for mitigating or relieving responsibility" (Scott and Lyman 1981:344–345).

For Scott and Lyman (1981:348) the crucial distinction between excuses and justifications is that in the former case the individual accepts that the behaviour in question is wrong, while in the latter case he or she "asserts its positive value in the face of a claim to the contrary." In addition to Sykes and Matza's (1957:667–669) techniques of neutralization ("denial of injury," "denial of victim," "condemnation of condemners," "denial of responsibility," and "appeal to loyalties"), they include self-fulfillment and sad tale accounts within their category of justifications. Self-fulfillment accounts justify behaviour through the rationale that the act is not wrong if it corresponds with the actor's notion of what is necessary to his or her self-fulfillment, whereas "The sad tale is a selected (often distorted) arrangement of facts that highlight an extremely dismal past, and thus explain the individual's present state" (Scott and Lyman 1981:349). Below,

I critically apply Scott and Lyman's (1981) notions of justifications and excuses, as well as Sykes and Matza's (1957) techniques of neutralization, in analysing informants' accounts of their experiences with alternative therapies. Further, I argue that the concept of retrospective reinterpretation of biographies can also be used to shed new light on how people who use alternative therapies reduce the stigma associated with their participation in alternative forms of health care.

ALTERNATIVE THERAPY USE AS DEVIANT BEHAVIOUR

The language used in the literature to describe alternative therapies has been and remains largely derogatory and pejorative. For example, consistently and over time, alternative therapies have been styled unconventional, nonconventional, unorthodox (Dunfield 1996); unscientific and unproven (Feigen and Tiver 1986); "fuzzy stuff" (Monson 1995:170); or "deviant forms of health service" (Cassee 1970:391). One extreme example concerns Leech's (1999:1) pronouncement that alternative therapies are "snake oil [which] belongs in the last century, not this or the next." Even when authors attempt neutrality through the use of concepts such as complementary therapy and/or medicine, they still imply a slur against alternative therapy by calling allopathic approaches conventional (Vincent and Furnham 1996) or regular medicine (Furnham and Smith 1988). For example, while she uses the term alternative medicine, Monson (1995:168) refers to allopathic health care as "proper orthodox medicine," implying that alternative therapies are unorthodox and improper. That allopathic medicine is assumed by many to be normative health care and that alternative therapies are not, is something the people who took part in this research are well aware of. For example, when I asked Pam to define alternative therapy, she said, "It's not going with the *norm* of the medical area that we have known for ever and ever. So anything that's not right there in the *straight* and *narrow* is going to be alternative" (emphases mine).

However, there is more to the deviant identities incurred through the use of alternative therapies than merely the "courtesy stigma" derived from participation in marginalized forms of health care (Goffman 1963:30). People who use alternative approaches to healing are seen as deviant in their own right. Their designation as deviant is less surprising in dated examples from the literature. For instance, over forty years ago, Cobb (1958:283) asserted that "There are four categories of patients who seek non-medical treatment. There are the miracle seekers, the uninformed, the restless ones, and the straw graspers." Yet, the labelling of alternative therapy use as deviant behaviour has continued over time. For example, decades later, Northcott (1994:498) restates Cobb's depiction of the user of alternative therapies in suggesting that these people may be "uneducated, ignorant, superstitious, gullible; hypochondriacs with psychosomatic problems ... motivated by fear [or] grasping at straws." Eight years later, Murray and Shepherd (1993:987) cite Furnham and Smith's (1988) contention that people who use alternative therapies are to be found amongst the chronically disturbed, citing the "relatively high frequency of psycho-social problems and affective disorders" diagnosed amongst the users of alternative therapies. Other authors characterize the users of alternative therapies as "naive" or unrealistic (Johnson 1999:230; Miller et al. 1998; Moenkhoft et al. 1999); and while Moore et al. (1985:28) assert that the people they studied are not "cranks," the implication is that they are not cranks because they haven't "lost faith in conventional medicine," not because there is nothing deviant about being a user of alternative therapies. More important from a symbolic interactionist perspective, however, is that all of the people who took part in this research had stories to tell of being labelled deviant for their use of alternative health care.[1]

Notwithstanding the continued popularity of these therapies and Sharma's (1993:15) claim that "It will not be long before the term 'alternative'—with its connotations of ... deviant activity—will no longer be appropriate," all informants have been subject to varying degrees of stigmatization for their use of alternative forms of health and healing. For instance, in response to various forms of the question, "How do others, your family and friends, react to your use of alternative therapies?," all informants had anecdotes to tell about how they had been ridiculed, embarrassed, patronized, and/or reacted to in an aggressive manner for their participation in alternative forms of health care. For example, in speaking about family members' reactions to her use of alternative therapies, Marie said, "They patronized you. 'Oh well this is a phase she's going through and then we can all have a good laugh about it.'" In addition to being patronized, several informants told stories of how they had been labelled "weird" by friends and family. Natalie told me friends "think I'm weird but that's OK. I had one person say: 'Are you a witch?' and I said: 'Well if I am I'm a good one or a kind one anyway.'" And Jenny described how an acquaintance thought she was weird because she used alternative approaches to healing:

This one person that I remember talking to about these courses that I've just taken recently in meditation and emotional healing said: 'Oh weird Californian stuff.' That was the reaction. Sometimes the response was generally obnoxious, aggressive, intrusive.

In Lindsay's case it was her boyfriend, as well as the parents of her equestrian students, who labelled her deviant for using acupuncture:

They think I'm a little weird. I run into it an awful lot; people think I'm a little strange. My boyfriend, for instance: he thought I was really, really strange when I started having the acupuncture done. You know [in a sarcastic tone]: 'What are you going to do next?' getting all [hums the theme song from The Twilight Zone].

Other informants told me of how friends, family members, health care professionals, and co-workers questioned their judgement or mental competency for their use of alternative therapies. For instance, in telling me about her friends' reaction to her disclosure that she uses alternative therapies, Betty said this: "It wasn't a case of laughing; in that case it almost went into an anger, or [they would say] 'Betty I can't believe, I never dreamed that you would be sucked into that.'" And Marie told me, "Some of [my friends] wrote me off as being a real crackpot: 'She's flipped, she's lost it, she's really gone off the deep end.' A few of them had stated it exactly that way." In addition to being labelled "flaky," Laura told me how her family saw her as an alternative health zealot: "They think it's really flaky or really fanatical. Like people who are into that kind of thing are fanatics about it." In Lorraine's case, her husband felt she had been hoodwinked: "So his thinking is: 'No, this is all a sham or a scam.'"

Furthermore, Yates et al. (1993:214) note that in the eyes of the medical profession the users of alternative therapies may be seen as "easily misled by false claims for unproven remedies." Similarly, participants in this research told me of how they had been depicted as gullible and/or naive by health care professionals. For example, Pam described how her child's doctor felt she was being duped by her naturopath: "The paediatrician, he did admit, he said, 'I'm very scientific, straight and narrow,' and he felt that we were being taken for a ride." Finally, Greg's co-workers labelled him gullible for his use of homeopathy and herbal remedies:

You just picked up on different ways that this stuff is flaky. Oh yeah, people will think that you're just—you'll get the rolling of eyes. At my place at work for a while I was the guy with the little funny bottles because I'd turn up with Echinacea or something like that and it was amazing to see what kind of a reaction I got out of taking out these small tincture bottles and putting a couple of drops under my tongue. [They'd say] 'Hey what is that? Can I get in on it?' and then I'd explain it to them and they'd say [in a sarcastic tone] 'So you think these work, do you?'

The particular type of deviant label applied to these people—flaky, weird, and/or gullible—did not vary by type of therapy used by informants. Neither did a pattern emerge between type of therapy and the instance or frequency of labelling, suggesting that it is the designation of alternative, rather than the specifics of a therapy, that leads others to label the individual as deviant. To illustrate, both Pam, who uses naturopathy, and Betty, who participates in crystal healing, are both labelled gullible, even though naturopathy was in the final stages of being regulated at the time these interviews took place. Furthermore, while Natalie is labelled a witch for her use of the results system, Marie is labelled gullible, without any connotations of the occult, for using *reiki*, a therapy employing comparable therapeutic techniques and sharing similar aspects of healing ideology. While these findings may seem surprising, social legitimation of a particular therapy did not necessarily protect these informants from being labelled deviant. As Greg put it, "I still come across people who are wary of chiropractors." His experience is noteworthy, as chiropractic treatment is the most established alternative therapy in Canada (Saks 1997a). While I found no relationship between informant experiences of being labelled and the type of therapy used, the instance and frequency of the labelling of these informants is shaped by the particular social context in which the interaction takes place. For example, two informants told me of how they had been labelled deviant for their use of alternative therapies within the context of Christian religious institutions. Hanna, who practices yoga, had this to say:

I forget, because I'm in an environment where we all basically believe in the same thing, but in the past I know it happened quite a few times. I worked in a church. I've had people I've helped, but when their ministers found out they told them to stop doing yoga immediately, even though it is benefiting them.

Betty, who uses *reiki*, crystal healing, and psychic healing, all therapeutic approaches with metaphysical underpinnings, told me this: "As I say, with the church [I used to belong to], as beautiful as they were, they were very against it. It never dawned on me I should never mention anything about the psychic to a minister, but obviously I shouldn't."

MANAGING THE STIGMA OF USING ALTERNATIVE THERAPIES

The people who spoke with me live with discreditable identities which they must manage (Goffman 1963). According to Goffman (1963), the difference between *discredited* and *discreditable* identities is that the latter depends on the degree to which individuals can reduce stigma by controlling disclosure of their deviant identity. Likewise, the literature shows that people who use alternative therapies make efforts to conceal their use from others, especially doctors (Montbriand and Laing 1991; Perlman et al. 1999; Ramsay et al. 1999). For instance, Eisenberg et al. (1993) found that over 70 percent of patients do not discuss their use of alternative therapies with their physicians, and Sharma (1992:55) reports that "interviewees expressed a positive concern that their GP should not find out about it, fearing ridicule or disapproval." Consistent with these findings, several of the people who participated in this research told me that they do not discuss their use of alternative therapies with their physicians. In Grace's words,

> I sort of went underground. I didn't tell [my doctor] what I was doing and I just sort of went ahead and I thought, 'Let's keep him happy and keep my medical plan happy, because I get a disability. I won't say anything. I will play the game.' I didn't tell him what I had done.

Nor would they readily disclose their use of alternative therapies to family, friends or acquaintances. According to Betty, "So at that point I thought, OK, there will be no more mention of it. With a lot of people, up until fairly recently, you'd be surprised how closed-mouthed I have been until I knew who I could talk to and who could be trusted and who couldn't." And while Nora felt comfortable discussing her use of alternative therapies with intimates, she is careful to whom else she discloses her participation in these forms of health care. She said:

> I'm pretty cautious about it, to be honest with you. I mean, people that are

friends that I socialize with, as opposed to acquaintances, my friends know that that's what I am more likely to do, something herbal or homeopathic or naturopathic, and they don't have a problem with it at all as far as I can tell; but I'm pretty cautious even with my friends, and especially with acquaintances, to say, 'Well, have you ever thought about such and such?'

Informants who practised alternative therapies were also reluctant to disclose their activities to others. For example, Lorraine suggested that I interview her friend Betty, who is a *reiki* practitioner. She said, "Betty and I travelled everywhere together because neither one of us knew what we wanted to specialize in. Now she has gone the healer route." However, when Betty and I spoke, she declined to identify herself in this way. I had noticed that she had a massage table in a room in her house and asked her if she was a *reiki* therapist. In an evasive tone she replied, "Oh no. I like to do my own thing and I do my thing on myself and on my husband." Lorraine suggested that Betty did not disclose her status as a practitioner because she charged people for *reiki* treatments without declaring the income she earned on her taxes. Another informant, Nora, also declined to identify herself as a practitioner but, in her case, the concern was fear of harassment and prosecution by the Canadian Medical Association (CMA) for practising medicine without a licence:

If somebody says I'm having a really hard time I can suggest some things, but there's also the reality that the Canadian Medical Association really doesn't like you to diagnose without a licence, diagnosing and prescribing, and I'm really sensitive to that around herbs. I'm a practitioner in some of these things in that I do work on myself, I use certain techniques and non-allopathic things for myself, for my animals when it's appropriate. I can suggest things for people but I'm very aware that the Canadian Medical Association has a real thing about it, and they also have the law on their side these days. I have no certificates. If I have ever made a tea up for anyone, and I've never charged them, I often ask if people will replace the herb for me; or if it was something that I would have to go and buy, then I say 'You go buy it and I'll mix it up in proportions,' and that's because I think there needs to be an exchange of some kind. But it is not my business, it is not my profession. It's what I choose to do and am willing to do to help people, but the medical associations are very pro-prietary around what is theirs. I'm quite conscious of that.

Illustrative of Goffman's (1963:42) classic phrasing, "To display or not to display; to tell or not to tell; to let on or not to let on; to lie or not to lie; and in each case, to whom, how, when, and where," these people are exercising caution in deciding with whom they will discuss their use or practice of alternative forms of health care. They said things like: "There were many situations where I would just not tell people [new acquaintances]. In many cases I just wouldn't mention it or talk about it in the first place or where I felt that maybe I was being ridiculed" (Jenny); "I'm a little bit cautious. I mean, even in terms of my own family I was truly the odd ball out and I would be very cautious when I would go to visit my family" (Trudy).

When managing disclosure is not an option, people may use humour as a method of reducing stigma (Davis 1961; Goffman 1963). For instance, Natalie told me, "I just laugh it off. I say: 'Well, we all have different ways of helping ourselves.'" And Brenda said, "With my doctor I don't really debate it, he's a cynical man. He always laughs at me and I always joke around with him about it." While informants used humour as a means of coping with stigma, this mode of stigma management attained varying degrees of success. For example, Lorraine described how she and her friends use humour with her husband; however, this has done little to lessen his negative appraisal of alternative therapies and those who use them:

> As much as my husband is exposed to this, let's say 80 percent of his life
> is exposed to my friends and I and this other world, we'll often tease and
> one of us will say: 'Let me do your feet Bob, let me heal you' [and he'll say
> angrily] 'Get away from me.'

Accounting for Stigma

In addition to managing disclosure and using humour, many of the people I spoke with used a variety of different types of *accounts* as linguistic devices for coping with the stigma they incur through their use of alternative therapies. These accounts take three forms: *the mistaken identity account*, the *ignorance of others account*, and accounts that make use of retrospective reinterpretation of biography as a means of reducing stigma—the *biographical account*. In the *mistaken identity account* the individual attributes his or her deviant identity to mistaken impressions made by others. For example, some informants managed stigma by giving accounts in which they claim they are not like the stereotype they perceive others hold, which assumes users of alternative therapies are cult-like fanatics out to convert non-believers. Others must certainly be mistaken if they identify them in this way. For example Roger said, "I don't make a point of proselytizing anything particularly," which Scott echoed with, "I don't try and convince people of anything. I'm not out to convert people." Similarly, Laura claimed, "I certainly don't consider myself fanatical. I don't push my ideas on anybody else," and Hanna told me, "I'm not that awful about it, I don't force my opinions."

In the *ignorance of others account*, the person attributes his or her deviant status to ignorance on the part of those who would label them. For instance, Simon's and Hanna's accounts of how they had been labelled deviant both made reference to the general ignorance of the other: "You know ignorance in action is frightening to behold; people aren't knowledgeable about different things. When I first was into vitamins and herbals, they wondered" (Simon);"There's a lot of ignorance about natural things like yoga and reflexology; they don't realize it's a philosophy and not an actual religion" (Hanna). Such was the imperative to distance themselves from deviant status (Goffman 1963) that Lucy was one of the few informants whose account included any "desire to ... enlighten" the ignorant (Scott and Lyman 1981:350). When I asked Lucy what she did when she encountered a negative reaction to her use of alternative therapies, she said, "Well, I'll explain it to the best of my ability. If they want more answers, I'll recommend people who've got better answers, who've got the answers."

Stigma Management Via Retrospective Reinterpretation

The third type of account employed as a method of managing stigma by the people who took part in this research is the *biographical account*. This type of account is one in which these informants reinterpret aspects of their biographies in order to show a clear, linear progression towards the use of alternative forms of health care. While they are aware that others may label their use of these therapies as deviant behaviour, they are able to see it, and themselves, as normal within the context of their reinterpreted biographies. In other words, alternative therapy use is something toward which they had always been moving. To illustrate, when discussing their use of alternative health care, almost half of the people I spoke with cited their parents' use of home remedies as foreshadowing their current use of alternative therapies. For instance, Marie told me, "Home remedies, the natural way of doing things. Going all the way back to Mum's chicken soup. My mother was very old-fashioned in her ways." This was echoed by Jane:

> She was just into home remedies. My mother was a smoker and if you had earaches as a kid she used to blow smoke in my ear. She would make bread poultices if you had splinters and mustard plasters when you had colds. She had a remedy for everything.

Betty also had a story to tell about her mother's home remedies:

> My mum always tried to make nutritious meals. We had our vitamins, which I believe in now within common sense, but I have in my cupboard my vitamins. I remember mum trying to get a spoonful of cod liver oil down me. They always believed in some of these extra things.

Past occupational experiences were another aspect of personal biography that some informants reinterpreted to mesh with their current participation in alternative therapies. For instance, Lucy and Marie had both worked in the health care system in the past. In their accounts of their use of alternative health care, they reinterpreted these experiences to coincide with their current use of alternative therapies. Marie reinterpreted her duties as a podiatrist's assistant as a precursor to her present-day engagement in training to become a reflexologist:

> I had worked for a podiatrist when I first got out of high school and part of his treatment was that after he finished with the patient, his digging and cutting and scraping and gouging, the last thing was that I went in for five minutes and I massaged their feet so that they left on a really positive note and I always knew the importance of that.

Similarly, in her account, Lucy reinterpreted her experiences working in a hospital as seminal events that inevitably led her to become a user of alternative therapies. In her words, "Well, I had always realized that the medical field can only basically deal with disease. It has to be a bacteria of some kind. If it's a virus they're helpless in that category. I've worked in a number of hospitals so I was well aware of that."

What is significant about this type of account is that it entails a reinterpretation rather than a necessarily factual recounting of personal biography. In other words, we engage in "biographical work where old objects must be reconstituted or given new meaning" (Corbin and Strauss 1987:264). That the importance of these past experiences is something that is assigned through retrospective reinterpretation is exemplified in Natalie's words below. While she believes that her past experiences at work are connected to her present-day use of alternative approaches to healing, her account belies the fact that she has reinterpreted her past occupational experience to explain her current use of alternative therapies. She put it this way:

> I used to say as I was nursing, 'There's gotta be better ways than what the doctor's ordering here, pushing pills.' I kept thinking 'This just isn't necessary,' but how could I stop it? Even after I gave up nursing and worked in a hospital as a ward clerk, I could see prostate after prostate after prostate coming out and I'm thinking, 'This has got to be wrong but they're continuing and they're still doing it,' and I think 'No, there's got to be another way.' I know when I held people's hands when they were dying they always felt very peaceful and they told me so, *but I didn't know what I was doing.* (emphasis mine)

Moreover, when I initially asked people when they first used alternative therapies, their answers described events that took place sometime in their adult years. Yet when I later asked them what family health care was like when they were children, they began telling me anecdotes about their parents' use of home remedies. In telling these stories, they connected their parents' use of home remedies with their own current use of alternative therapies. That these accounts entailed retrospective reinterpretation is evidenced by the fact that the use of home remedies was something these informants' parents no doubt viewed as conventional rather than alternative, if only because at that time in history Canadian Medicare did not exist. Consequently, most Canadians employed home remedies as a form of self-care before resorting to paying for a physician (Heeney 1995). For example, Jane told me, "Not for check-ups; just if you were sick. We used to pay doctors for visits when I was very young until I was in my teens, until we had medical coverage."

Therefore, the accounts informants gave of their parents' use of home remedies are better understood as on-the-spot reinterpretation of their biographies in order to create a coherent, linear progression which explains their present-day use of alternative health care. For example, in looking back and recasting her biography, Nora speculated about a connection between her mother's use of home remedies and her current participation in alternative health care:

> I guess I always knew that there were ways to effect better health probably from way, way back in the dark ages when I was a little kid and my mother used to do home remedies. Sore throat, a flannel cloth soaking wet around your neck with a wool sock on that and tied at the back. *So probably that was my first experience of it.* (emphasis mine)

Randal also reinterpreted his mother's and grandmother's use of home remedies as an explanation for his present-day participation in alternative therapies: "This was stuff that my mother had taught me when I was a kid. *It was like a trigger.* Things that my godmother had taught me about how to pick the herbs in the forest" (emphasis mine). Brenda and Trudy also reinterpreted memories of their parents' use of folk and home remedies in light of their contemporary participation in alternative health care. Trudy told me, "My mom's approach, when I had worms, she ended up [using] onion and garlic. She knew exactly what to do. She obviously was in that mode [of alternative therapies]. We never put salt on our foods. *So I think it's just always been there*" (emphasis mine). And Brenda said,

> I think being from Poland my parents were also into home remedies. You know, poultices when I got bitten by a mosquito and herbal teas to this day and camomile. Always my parents, or at least my mother always had a keen interest and some information stayed with me. *I remember now.* (emphasis mine)

In addition to the ubiquitous stigma reduction techniques of managing disclosure and using humour, many of the people who took part in this research employed a variety of types of accounts as a means of coping with the stigma engendered through participation in alternative therapies. These accounts can be categorized into three types: the *mistaken identity account*, the *ignorance of others account*, and the *biographical account*. All three of these types of accounts share some similarities with one or another of the justificatory accounts and/or excuses described by Scott and Lyman (1981) and Sykes and Matza (1957). For example, *the ignorance of others* account is similar to Scott and Lyman's (1981:350) self-fulfillment account, where individuals justify their behaviour by "indicat[ing] a desire to ... enlighten what they considered to be the unenlightened establishment." However, the account invoked by these informants differs in that it is more concerned with pointing out the general ignorance of others than with any desire to enlighten. In this way the *ignorance of others account* is more analogous to Sykes and Matza's (1957:668) condemnation of condemners, where the individual attempts to deflect "attention from his [or her] deviant acts to the motives and behaviour of those who disapprove of his [or her] violation." Yet, again, this type of account differs from that described by Sykes and Matza's (1957), as the words used by these informants has more of a flavour of acceptance of the unavoidable ignorance of others than it does condemnation of others for their ignorance.

In much the same way, the *mistaken identity account* is consistent with some aspects of Scott and Lyman's (1981) self-fulfillment account and Sykes and Matza's (1957) condemnation of condemners, as the technique of stigma management in all three cases entails a shifting of the focus of attention away from the action and/or motives of the labelled and toward those of the labeller. Nonetheless, there remains a difference between them. While these informants' accounts do contain a depiction of the other as unenlightened, the unenlightened behaviour is understood as a mistake. Rather than condemning the other for being just as bad as they themselves are, these people see their use of these therapies as normal. Moreover, their accounts also render the other's actions as the epitome of normative behaviour; for as we all know, everybody makes mistakes. Notwithstanding what is distinctive about the ignorance of others and the mistaken identity accounts, the differences I have just sketched between them and the accounts described by Scott and Lyman (1981) and Sykes and Matza (1957), are merely differences of type. As Scott and Lyman (1981:345 f.n.10) themselves point out, their discussion of types of excuses is meant "to be taken as illustrative rather than as an exhaustive listing." However, in the biographical account I argue that there is a difference of theoretical import.

While the *biographical account* is also similar to Scott and Lyman's (1981) concept of the sad tale account in that both aim to minimize stigma through the reordering or reinterpretation of past life events, there is a significant difference between them. The biographical account differs in that it does not depend on a "distorted arrangement of facts that highlight an extremely dismal past" which compelled the individual to become deviant (Scott and Lyman 1981:349). In contrast, in the *biographical account* the past is rendered in neutral terms and is used as an *explanation*, rather than *justification*, for one's present-day use of alternative therapies. The *biographical account* represents an appeal to inevitability rather than the appeal to hard times invoked by the sad tale. This sense of inevitability contained within the biographical account suggests a superficial likeness with Scott and Lyman's (1981:345–347) notion of the "appeal to biological drives," a case where the individual attempts to excuse his or her deviant behaviour by asserting that it is the result of biological determinism and thus beyond his or her control.

However, the *biographical account* is different because it is an account in which the actor explains rather than justifies or excuses his or her acts. In other words, what is at issue for informants invoking the *biographical account*, is making sense of their actions through connecting the past with the present. They are normalizing both past and present behaviour, in contrast to excusing or justifying, by pinpointing an event in the past responsible for deviance in the present. In this way the biographical account enables the actor to better avoid reinforcement of the deviant label characteristic of secondary deviance (Lemert 1951). Therefore, what is most significant is that these accounts differ because they are not justifications or excuses: they are explanatory accounts that rest upon an *appeal to biographic consistency*. They are these informants' attempts to make linear biographical sense of their use of alternative therapies, to normalize their participation in these forms of healing rather than an attempt to excuse or justify it.

In closing, one must point out that there is a practical significance to these informants' use of retrospective reinterpretation as a means of stigma management. Namely, all of the people who took part in this research told me of benefits they derive through their use of alternative therapies. However, the stigma attached to alternative forms of health care poses a potential constraint on their use of these therapies. Nonetheless, through the use of retrospective reinterpretation of biography, they are able to overcome this barrier and are thereby able to access therapies they believe are beneficial to them.

NOTES

1. I found a similar pattern of stigmatization among users of alternative and complementary therapies who took part in research I conducted in the UK. Almost all of them reported instances of being labelled deviant for their participation in alternative and complementary approaches, despite the greater acceptance of these forms of health care in the UK relative to North America (Low 2001b).

Conclusion[1]

This book emerged out of a qualitative study of lay participation in alternative health care. Through a symbolic interactionist analysis of the experiences of the people who spoke with me, I have argued that objectivist definitions of alternative therapies are inherently problematic. However, we can make meaningful reference to these forms of health care from a subjectivist perspective and with attention to social context, to the nature of the everyday experience of these therapies, and to the claims various groups of individuals, including lay people, make about these approaches to health and healing. I have also demonstrated that people who use alternative health care are not marked by particular characteristics; rather, they are individuals who reflect the general population.

The people who took part in this research began using alternative therapies through a variety of different points of *entrée* into alternative health care networks made up of alternative practitioners and other lay users of alternative therapies. Acknowledging that these therapies permeate the health care system means that the only fruitful distinction we can make between forms of therapy is whether or not they are regulated in some fashion. Furthermore, how these people experience their alternative health care networks required a reconceptualization of the health care system to account for the fact that accessing alternative therapies can be a difficult process at times. However, despite the constraints on access these informants experienced, a significant finding is that they were also able to engage in experimentation with alternative therapies in ways they are unable to do with allopathic health care.

In general, the people who spoke with me were not seeking forms of health care that conformed to alternative ideologies of health and healing they espoused prior to their participation in these therapies. Rather, they sought out alternative approaches in order to address health problems, both personal and physical, for which they hitherto had found no solution. Thus the use of alternative therapies is no different than any other form of health-seeking behaviour. Moreover, it is better understood through the generic social process of problem-solving, rather than through the push/pull dynamics of particular motivating factors.

While these people were not shopping for an ideology when they first sought out alternative therapies, participation in these approaches to health care led to their adoption of alternative health and healing beliefs—beliefs that inform their alternative models of health and healing. They gave meaning to their alternative model of health through what they see as the distinctly alternative conceptual categories of holism, balance and control. For these people, to be healthy is to be engaged in the process of healing, which they see as a categorically different understanding of health to that embodied in allopathic notions of health, illness, and disease. In contrast, they gave meaning to the components of their alternative model of healing by making constant reference to what they understand as the negative standard of biomedicine. While these informants value the differences they see between alternative and allopathic approaches to health and health care, critical analysis of their alternative model of health reveals that it fares no better than the biomedical model where the charge of blaming the individual for problems of ill health is concerned. Rather, their alternative model of health is equally reductionist in turning attention away from the social production of illness and disease. In addition, the benefits to health and self these people attribute to their participation in alternative therapies are only available to those with the resources (i.e., time and money) to pursue them.

Finally, I have shown how espousal of alternative ideologies of health and healing can have a profound impact on individuals' subjective perceptions of self. These ideologies affected informants' identities in two significant ways. Some of them became so committed to their new health beliefs that they began the process of becoming alternative practitioners themselves. For others the impact was more extensive: the ideology contained within the alternative model of health and healing became a mechanism through which they transformed their personal identities for the better. In particular, it became the means by which they are able to construct a sense of self that is healthy, even in the presence of biomedically defined disease and infirmity. Nonetheless, in addition to the positive impact on self they experience, their use of these therapies also means that they are vulnerable to the label of deviant health seeker, thus requiring that they manage the stigma conferred through participation in these therapies.

IMPLICATIONS FOR HEALTH POLICY

The findings from this research have implications for the formation of health policy in Canada. In particular, they are relevant to the debates surrounding the possibilities for, and consequences of, integration of alternative with allopathic approaches to health and healing, as well as the inclusion of alternative therapies within Canadian Medicare. To illustrate, a variety of factors indicate that inclusion of alternative and complementary therapies within Canada's public health care provision is a potential reality. For instance, the vast popularity of these approaches to health and healing among Canadians alone would encourage the extension of Medicare to cover alternative and complementary therapies. According to Tataryn and Verhoef (2001:VII.97), "increasing consumer utilisation and demand" constitute "upward pressure" towards integration and has already affected many "levels of health care [and] ... clinical and institutional initiatives." Furthermore, if Canadian health policy makers heed the World Health Organisation's (WHO 2000:17) conclusion that a key measure of the success of health care systems is responsiveness, where responsiveness is defined as the degree to which health care systems "respond to people's expectations," lay desire for alternative therapies should foster inclusion under public health insurance in Canada.

Moreover, there are some signs that the medical profession's traditional resistance to alternative forms of healing is eroding. For instance, Balon et al. (2001a:IV.49) assert that "leaders from both conventional medicine and complementary/alternative practitioners see greater integration as necessary and desirable." There is also evidence of the increasing adoption of alternative approaches to health and alternative therapeutic techniques by the medical community (Achilles et al. 1999; Tataryn and Verhoef 2001; Northcott 1994). In addition, some Canadian medical schools are beginning to integrate training in alternative and complementary therapies into their curriculum (Tataryn and Verhoef 2001). For instance, 89 percent of the eight medical schools, and 90 percent of the twenty-eight nursing schools, Achilles et al. (1999:231) surveyed, responded that they offered courses that "include information on alternative and complementary therapies;" and Balon et al. (2001a:IV.50) state that 38 percent of Canadian medical schools ... now offer stand alone courses in complementary medicine." Similarly, alternative practitioners are increasingly engaged in the process of becoming recognized legitimated professionals requiring incorporation of biomedical paradigms of health and healing within their educational regimes (Boon 1998; Saks 1995; Sharma 1993). Further, some Canadian health care professionals "make referrals to complementary and alternative practitioners," albeit almost always to chiropractors (Tataryn and Verhoef 2001:VII.98). Similarly, while the people who took part in this research were not referred *per se*, several of them did access alternative therapies through recommendations made by their physicians.

Thus, it can be argued that the boundaries between allopathic and alternative approaches to health care are beginning to blur. For instance, Tataryn and Verhoef (2001:94–98) argue that both allopathic and alternative health care stress preventative and patient-centred care. They further assert that nursing and family medicine "share assumptions related to holistic care ... with complementary and alternative modalities." In addition, the emphasis on self-control within these informants' model of health resonates with general cultural notions of health. For example, Crawford (1984) argues that there are two general lay concepts of health in contemporary culture: health as control and health as release. Health as control defines health as a status achieved by "self discipline, self denial, and will power;" and health as release, while seeming to reject the constraints of the control model, highlights "the psychological capacity for not worrying," hinging on an individual's self-control of stress (Crawford 1984:66,82). The alternative model of health's insistence that individuals control their minds, lifestyles, and, in particular, stress, makes this model entirely consistent with a general cultural understanding of health. Hence, to the degree that allopathic and alternative paradigms can be harmonized, the integration of alternative therapies within Medicare will be facilitated. More precisely, to the extent that *allopathy* becomes more *alternative* and *alternative* becomes more *allopathic*, alternative health care could be said to be integrated into Canadian public health care provision.

Furthermore, certain alternative or complementary therapies are already available under Medicare. For example, chiropractic and naturopathic treatment is provided under the public insurance programme in British Columbia; and Alberta, Saskatchewan, Manitoba, Ontario, and Quebec all allow some access to chiropractic under Medicare (Achilles et al. 1999). While very few alternative therapies are currently available under public health insurance in Canada, the presence of chiropractic and naturopathy could represent the thin edge of the wedge where inclusion of other alternative healing modalities are concerned.

Finally, there are a number of research initiatives focussing on alternative and complementary therapies that have been completed or are ongoing in Canada. Notably, Health Canada has funded and/or sponsored a number of these studies (Achilles et al. 1999). For instance, the Tzu Chi Institute has completed research on integrated health care and mapping of organizations that "deliver, educate, regulate, and support alternative and complementary" health care, among other projects and activities related to these approaches to health and healing (Achilles et al. 1999:244). The Calgary Research Centre for Alternative Medicine has completed case studies of alternative and complementary therapies, in addition to organizing several conferences on these forms of health care. They have also partnered with the federal government in the National Forum on Health and the Health Canada Expert Advisory Committee on Complementary Medicine (Achilles et al. 1999). Finally, but not exhaustively, Pawluch et al. (1998b) conducted research for Health Canada focussed on the use of complementary health care among people living with HIV/AIDS, and the York University Centre for Health Studies published a 1999 report for Health Canada documenting the "landscape in which complementary and alternative health care practices and therapies are provided ... from a national perspective" (Achilles et al. 1999:3).

While there is a certain amount of momentum towards integration of alternative and allopathic paradigms of health and healing, as well as the inclusion of alternative therapies within Medicare, there remain a number of significant barriers to overcome. To begin with, establishing the efficacy and safety of alternative and complementary forms of health care is argued to be crucial to the inclusion of these approaches within public health care provision (Achilles et al. 1999; Balon et al. 2001a; Crosby 1999; Ernst 1997; Ernst and Fugh-Berman 1999; House of Lords 2000:para 9.39; Tataryn and Verhoef 2001). However, a major constraint on inclusion is medical, scientific dominance over assessing the efficacy of alternative therapies. For example, many medical and health policy researchers argue that "only services for which there is convincing evidence of their benefits, preferably beyond the placebo effects and in referenced journals" should be provided by public health care (Crosby 1999; Ernst 1997; Ernst and Fugh-Berman 1999). Such assertions reveal a double standard inherent in the current drive to evaluate the efficacy of alternative and complementary health care. Namely, while it is true that the efficacy of the majority of these therapies has not been formally established, neither has the effectiveness of upwards of 85 percent of medical interventions (Balon et al. 2001a; Evans 1993; Rawsthorne et al. 1999; Smith 1991; Tataryn and Verhoef 2001). This double standard works against the inclusion of alternative therapies within Medicare.

In addition, there are substantial methodological problems inherent in assessing the efficacy of alternative and complementary approaches to health care which, moreover, "are not common issues among" allopathic therapeutic modalities (Achilles et al. 1999:249; Balon et al. 2001a; Tataryn and Verhoef 2001).[2] For instance, The Canadian Cancer Society has stated that it is "difficult for them to fit complementary and alternative therapies into the scientific paradigm of the National Cancer Institute of Canada." Nonetheless, the vast majority of authors concerned with the efficacy of alternative health care argue that medical scientific research designs are the only valid means of evaluating the effectiveness of these therapies.[3] For many of them, the randomized controlled trial (RCT) is the "gold standard" in research designs for these purposes.[4] Similarly, Walker and Anderson (1999:1615) assert that for alternative and complementary therapies "to be accepted by conventional practitioners, they will need to be evaluated using RCT and the results published in peer reviewed journals" held in esteem by scientists and conventional practitioners."[5] However, there is evidence that "a bias against publication" of studies of alternative therapies exists (Resch et al. 2000:166).

Moreover, the RCT method is ill equipped for the evaluation of alternative therapies (Balon et al. 2001a). For example, researchers have pointed out the difficulty of "securing agreement about standard forms of treatment," given that individualized treatment is an essential component of the means by which these approaches effect healing, according to the people I spoke with, alternative practitioners, and other lay users of alternative therapies (Lowenberg 1992; Jobst 2000; Meade et al. 1990:1431; Veal 1998). Nahin and Straus (2001) add that standardization is complicated by the fact that there are multiple schools of the same therapy in existence (i.e., Western versus Chinese schools of acupuncture) that have divergent beliefs about treatment regimes based on conflicting healing paradigms.

Also problematic in RCT assessment of the efficacy of alternative and complementary therapies are the issues of recruitment, randomization, and patient preferences (Fitter and Thomas 1997). For example, Walker and Anderson (1999:1615) argue that "Many CAM practitioners emphasize the need for a genuinely collaborative approach to clinical decision making" which means that randomization, for instance, "preclude[s] evaluating certain treatment under everyday conditions." Another problem in applying the RCT method to the assessment of these therapies concerns the preference for blinding in RCT designs (Hart 2001). For example, blinding is impossible with therapies such as therapeutic massage or chiropractic treatment where there is physical contact between therapist and client (Fitter and Thomas 1997; Nahin and Straus 2001; Walker and Anderson 1999). Moreover, trials making use of placebos or shams as a control are problematic because within alternative healing paradigms, placebos are "*catalysts* of the bioregulatory mechanisms" rather than shams (Birch 1997; Lowenberg 1992; Tonkin 1987:7, emphasis his).[6] Finally, RCTs typically select a single treatment modality for study, whereas many alternative and complementary therapies are complex interventions comprising a variety of healing techniques (Fitter and Thomas 1997; Hamilton and Betchel 1996; Nahin and Straus 2001). For instance, naturopathy, one of the therapeutic approaches used by the people who took part in this research, typically includes several alternative therapies, such as homeopathy, herbal remedies, massage, and yoga, as well as nutrition and lifestyle counselling, among other therapeutic modalities (Clarke 1996; Northcott 1994).

An additional problem in the positivistic assessment of the efficacy of these forms of health care is that despite claims that allopathic and alternative approaches are beginning to converge, there remain irreconcilable differences between alternative and allopathic paradigms of disease and treatment. According to Calmels (1999:129), Chinese "acupuncture ... takes into account the influence of ... 'Universal Harmony.'" Similarly, many of the participants in this research emphasized the role played by universal energy in healing; however, neither "are usually ... taken into consideration by scientific medicine" (Calmels 1999:129). Moreover, Murphy (2000) argues that scientific research designs fail to take account of the states of mind of the client and practitioner as a form of treatment modality in and of itself, despite the fact that it is a key component of the model of alternative healing espoused by the people who took part in this research.

Another potential barrier to the inclusion of these therapies within mainstream health care provision concerns their safety. Some authors warn that *all* alternative and complementary therapies are potentially dangerous to the degree that they detour people away from scientifically proven medical care (Ernst 1997; Feigen and Tiver 1986; Gottlieb 2001, emphasis mine). Similarly, a great deal of the literature on the efficacy of alternative and complementary therapies is concerned with the possible dangers posed by participation in these forms of health care.[7] For example, while they cite no evidence of side effects in using these therapies to treat attention-deficit hyperactivity disorder, Stubberfield et al. (1999:452) caution that "medical practitioners ... should be aware ... of the possible adverse effects of these" forms of health care. In particular, there is concern over the iatrogenic potential of acupuncture as well as harmful interactions between medication and herbal remedies or vitamins (Eisenberg et al., cited in Bender 1999:41; Ernst 2000a, 1997).[8] However, while research on alternative and complementary therapies is ongoing in Canada, "much research about complementary and alternative health care" remains to be done (Balon et al. 2001a:IV:49; Tataryn and Verhoef 2001). Compounding this problem is that there is insufficient funding for such research (Tataryn and Verhoef 2001). As one physician (Achilles et al. 1999:217) interviewed said, "research dollars are zero."

There is also continued resistance from the medical community to both the regulation of alternative practitioners and the inclusion of alternative and complementary therapies within Medicare. In particular, physicians express "concern over loss of professional identity and the potential fiscal and professional impact of sharing the consumer health care market with other professions" (Tataryn and Verhoef 2001:VII.99). Another effect of this resistance is that physicians, in general, lack information about these therapies and are without a perspective through which to understand them (Achilles et al. 1999). While there is some recognition by medical professionals that physicians need to have at least an elementary understanding of the alternative therapies their patients use so they are better able to counsel them (Ernst 2000a), many physicians have little knowledge of these forms of health care (Balon et al. 2001a; Perlman et al. 1999). Likewise, authors argue that "the education of many complementary and alternative practitioners includes too little foundation in conventional approaches ... to enable effective integrative care" (Balon et al. 2001a:IV.50). Both physician efforts at professional boundary maintenance and their lack of knowledge about these therapies are evidenced by the lack of truly complementary health care experienced by the people I spoke with.

Furthermore, continued stigmatization of lay users of alternative therapies, including the people who took part in this research, works against inclusion and is reflective of the persistent marginal status of these forms of health care (Saks 1995). Finally, what might be the single most important factor in mitigating against inclusion of alternative and complementary therapies within Medicare is provincial and federal government concerns over costs, specifically, fears that inclusion of alternative therapies would result in "increased service options translating into escalating reimbursement and operating costs" (Tataryn and Verhoef 2001:99). This is an issue that was noted by some of the people I spoke with, among them Nora:

> I mean if people were using homeopathy then they're not, I mean, I don't and the last time I saw my doctor was two years ago. She said: 'I wouldn't see you as a major [cost] factor in the health care system based on the number of times you see me.' What I do is at my cost. I pay for them and save the medical system a huge amount of money, so do other people like myself.

Putting aside the factors that work against integration of alternative with allopathic approaches, and the inclusion of alternative therapies within Medicare, both integration and inclusion would have a number of positive consequences for Canadians engaged in health-seeking behaviour. For instance, the people I spoke with would welcome inclusion of alternative therapies under public health insurance to the extent that it would help them overcome the barriers they face in accessing these forms of health care. These barriers include a lack of financial resources, a lack of information about alternative and complementary therapies, a lack of support from health care professionals, and stigma.

That a lack of financial resources constrains access to these therapies is evidenced by the fact that Canadians spend between 1.8 billion and 3.8 billion dollars on alternative health care strategies annually (Angus Reid 1998; de Bruyn 2001:II.23). A lack of information about what kinds of therapies are available is another significant barrier to access for people who would like to use alternative therapies. While some therapists are members of professional bodies and/or are listed in directories or registers, most of the alternative and complementary therapists consulted by the people who took part in this study are not. Similarly, medical and other health care professionals are unlikely to be able to provide information about these therapies. In addition, the labelling of people who use alternative therapies as deviant both limits their access to these therapies and mitigates against achieving complementary health care. To the degree that their allopathic health care professionals collude in this labelling process, inclusion of these therapies within Canada's mainstream health care provision would reduce the stigma associated with participation in alternative therapies and encourage physicians to be supportive of their use, thus improving access. Likewise, inclusion would remove the barriers of cost and improve access to information about these approaches to health and healing.

Finally, inclusion of alternative and complementary therapies within Medicare would show that health policymakers are responsive to the needs and desires of Canadians (WHO 2000). Furthermore, integration of allopathic with alternative healing approaches and inclusion of alternative therapies within Medicare would enable the people who took part in this research to address health problems for which they found no redress prior to their participation in alternative forms of healing. Finally, given these informants' alternative model of health's emphases on prevention, and its orientation towards chronic conditions, integration of alternative and allopathic healing paradigms would also positively affect population health and enable the Canadian health care system to better cope with the incidence of chronic illness.

Notwithstanding these positive consequences, it is important to consider the ways in which integration of alternative and allopathic healing ideology or inclusion of alternative therapies within mainstream health care provision may not necessarily be entirely desirable. For instance, Glik (1988:1205) argues that "Attempts to 'medicalize' healing practices by employing them in clinical contexts may rob these practices of their effectiveness." To illustrate, Margolin et al. (cited in Bender 1999:42) state that submitting alternative and complementary therapies to the RCT research design requires practitioners

> to undertake a fundamental conceptual shift from a view of patients as requiring individualized treatment that may vary at each session to one in which trial participants are regarded as members of an equivalent class, defined by the diagnosis, who all will be given a standard prescribed treatment.

Such standardization would result in reduced efficacy of alternative therapies according to these informants' alternative model of healing, under which the effectiveness of a therapy is due in part to individualized treatment regimes. In particular, it would likely divest their alternative model of health of its power to heal the self, one that lies in their perception of the distinctiveness of their alternative definition of health from biomedical understandings.

Inclusion of these therapies within Medicare would also interfere with how the people I spoke with use alternative therapies by constraining their ability to self-prescribe, experiment, and dabble in alternative therapies, as these approaches to health and healing would then be subject to the same gatekeeping practices as allopathic interventions. Furthermore, to the extent to which inclusion depends on scientific evidence of efficacy and medically rational explanation, some alternative or complementary therapies that "work" may remain "unproven." For example, Jobst (2000:295) states that "The mechanism of action of homeopathic potencies remains inexplicable according to the current biomedical paradigm," despite the fact that lay people find it an effective treatment (Taylor et al. 2000). Moreover, the Lords Select Committee report (House of Lords 2000:9.39) recommends that "only CAM therapies with an adequate evidence base in their favour should be considered for" inclusion within public health care, and that only acupuncture, chiropractic, herbal medicine, and osteopathy have established such evidence to any degree. It is noteworthy, therefore, that many of the therapies used by these informants, including those they found most effective, are not found amongst those endorsed by the Western medical community.

Finally, among the potential negative consequences of the efforts of alternative practitioners to become regulated professionals is that they may no longer have the power to challenge institutionalized biomedicine. Furthermore, the integration of alternative and allopathic approaches could rob the former of its ability to serve as a catalyst for innovation within mainstream health care provision. In Stambolovic's (1996:603) words, "it is so important to nurture heresy's imperfection, [especially] those parts that leave room for inquiry and change."

Given the potential for negative consequences of inclusion and integration, policymakers should be aware that lay experience of alternative approaches to health and healing dictate that, first and foremost, care should be taken that integration of alternative and allopathic healing approaches does not become manifest in the medicalization of alternative ideologies of health and healing. Due care should also be taken that regulation of alternative therapies reflect these individuals' desire to take control of their healing process, which they accomplish, in part, through the freedom to experiment with alternative therapies. For example, in discussing a proposed bill that would include Vitamin C under the controlled substances act, Nora told me this:

> If they outlawed alternative medicine, would you stop using it? Would you strategize around how to get access to things that will become illegal...? I mean there's lobbying.... I'd break the law if it was against the law because I think my health is my business and because it might be that my whole life or my whole being depended on that. It has to do with my health, so I really do think that when the state interferes and things like that it is never about protection; it's about control.

Similarly, where assessing the safety of these therapies is concerned, policymakers should note that "the truth is that most therapies have direct risks and side effects" (Ernst 1997:43, emphasis mine). For instance, Odsberg et al. (2001:17) reports that evidence of iatrogenic effects from acupuncture "in relation to the number of practitioners is very low, especially if a comparison is made with traditional pharmacological therapy." Some authors, while agreeing that ensuring the safety of all therapies is important and necessary, see the undue focus on safety in studies of alternative and complementary therapies as scaremongering, especially when compared to the rates of iatrogenic effects in medical interventions (Illich 1975). For example, in response to the headline: *Patient Dies of Alternative Cancer Remedy,* in the *British Medical Journal* (Gottlieb 2001), Lade (2000:1491) wrote as follows: "Why not make a headline such as: *10 000 people died from complications of cancer this week even though they had the standard conventional treatment.*" Further, the people I spoke with, and lay people in general, are confident that their alternative therapies are non-iatrogenic and safe to use, especially when compared to allopathic forms of treatment (Boon et al. 1999; Boutin et al. 2000; Johnson 1999; Low 2001b). Therefore, Health Canada would do better to broaden its scope to address the safety of all interventions, whether alternative or allopathic, rather than focus exclusively on the safety of alternative therapies (Balon et al. 2001a).

In addition, regarding the efficacy of these therapies, policymakers need to widen the boundaries of what is considered valid evidence of the effectiveness of a therapy to include more than just methods consistent with the natural science model. For instance, Rawsthorne et al. (1999:1302) argue as follows:

Some physicians may view that alternative medicine is simply a placebo. However, placebos have been shown to be associated with considerable response rates among patients with active disease. This proves that therapies lacking obvious scientific bases for effecting disease improvement may nonetheless work.

Therefore, Health Canada would be wise to adopt an approach such as that advocated by a small minority of authors who suggest the benefits of using more than one type of evidence. For example, Barton (2000:256) suggests a "flexible approach in which randomised controlled trials and observation studies have complementary roles," and White and Ernst (2001:112) allow that uncontrolled clinical trials can be used "as 'pilot' or 'feasibility' studies to guide subsequent controlled research."[9] Further, Hamilton and Bechtel (1996:7) advocate triangularization of methods as a means of "strengthening the trustworthiness of research findings by using multiple theoretical frameworks and sources of data." And Nahin and Straus (2001:163) conclude that "Although randomised controlled trials are the accepted standard of clinical research, [the National Centre for Alternative and Complementary Medicine] values other types of high quality research, including careful observational studies" and research conducted through interdisciplinary teams using a variety of forms of evidence.

From the perspective of the lay user of alternative therapies, greater weight is accorded to lay referral systems and individual experiences of efficacy over medical referral and expert validation in lay participation in these forms of health care (Low 2001b; Kacperek 1997; Boon et al. 1999; Gray et al. 1998). In general, the conceptual models of assessing efficacy employed by lay people are complex; they are made up of different combinations of elements of both alternative and allopathic healing ideology, and in these models, lay people assign greater weight to the role of subjective perceptions—over positivistic measures—in establishing the effectiveness of a therapy (Low 2001b). Moreover, lay people show a relative lack of interest in why something works (Low 2001b), suggesting a greater concern with outcomes than with mechanisms of action. A primary concern with outcomes is consistent with the current vogue in evidence-based medicine. Indeed, even the Lords Select Committee concluded that a lack of explanation for the efficacy of these therapies "should not be a barrier to acceptance by ... the medical profession" (Mills 2001:36). Therefore, any research strategy concerned with the inclusion of alternative approaches to health and healing within Medicare should accord a prominent place to lay perspectives on alternative therapies.

SUGGESTIONS FOR FUTURE RESEARCH

Canadian policy researchers have concluded that more research needs to be done prior to inclusion of alternative and complementary therapies within Canadian public health provision (Achilles 2001; Tataryn and Verhoef 2001). I would add that in particular, research on the efficacy of these therapies from the lay perspective is required. Very few studies have examined how lay people assess the effectiveness of the alternative and complementary approaches to health and healing they use. Furthermore, the bulk of this literature does little more than report that people believe that they derive a benefit from their participation in alternative and complementary therapies[10] and/or are highly satisfied with their experiences with these therapies.[11] While some researchers have engaged in deeper explanatory analysis of lay perspectives on the efficacy of alternative therapies, almost all are set in the US or UK context (Gray et al. 1998; Launsø 2000; Low 2001b; Stubberfield et al. 1999; Vincent et al.1995). Boon et al. (1999) and Gray et al. (1998) are among the very few authors who address the perspectives of Canadians regarding the effectiveness of alternative health care. Such research would provide us with a more holistic understanding of *what works* and also with better evidence to determine which therapies should be included within Medicare.

Another direction for future research concerns the following question: To what extent do alternative approaches to health and healing continue to constitute a challenge to biomedical dominance and thus serve as a catalyst for change within allopathic health care? For example, Schneirov and Geczik (1996) argue that the users of alternative therapies are members of a new social movement that presents an institutional challenge to bio-medicine, and Wolpe (1990:922) concludes that alternative practitioners serve as "gatekeepers of orthodox medicine" who have the freedom to experiment with new therapies which can then be incorporated into allopathic practice, thus expanding the range of therapeutic techniques available under public health care provision. However, Schneirov and Geczik (1996:638) also assert that participation in alternative approaches to health and healing constitutes a social network movement that is "submerged within everyday life rather than engaging in visible political activities that confront authorities." Moreover, Saks (1998:211) concludes that

> there is not as yet a postmodern profusion of heterogeneity so much as
> a new way of legitimating the continuing dominance of medical authority
> through a strategy based on incorporation and subordination, in face of
> the growing challenge from complementary approaches.

Therefore, research should track the influences of the movement towards integration of allopathic and alternative approaches to health and healing, in addition to the inclusion of alternative therapies within public health provision, to determine the effect of these processes on the potential of alternative therapies, as well as on the lay people and practitioners who use them, to continue to play an innovative and revolutionary role within the health care system.

NOTES

1. Portions of this chapter were previously published in the journal *Evidence-Based Integrative Medicine*(2003), 1(1):65–76.
2. See also Birch (1997); Calmels (1999); Fitter and Thomas (1997); Gadsby et al. (1997); Hamilton and Bechtel (1996); Hart (2001); Jobst (2000); Lindenmuth and Lindenmuth (2000); Long et al. (2000); Meade et al. (1990); Murphy (2000); Nahin and Straus (2001); Tonkin (1987); Veal (1998); and Walker and Anderson (1999).
3. See Barton (2000); Bender (1999); Bossuyt (2001); Calmels (1999); Critchley et al. (2000); Crosby (1999); Drew and Davies (2001); Ernst (2000a, 2000b, 1999, 1997); Ernst and Barnes (1998); Ernst and Fugh-Berman (1999); Gadsby et al. (1997); Leibovici (1999); Lewith et al. (2000); Taylor et al. (2000); Thomas and Fitter (1997); Vickers and Smith (1997); and Walker and Anderson (1999).
4. See Barton (2000); Bossuyt (2001); Drew and Davies (2001); Ernst (2000a,1999, 1997); Ernst and Barnes (1998); Ernst and Fugh-Berman (1999); Gadsby et al. (1997); Taylor et al. (2000); Thomas and Fitter (1997:94); and Walker and Anderson (1999).
5. The few authors who critique the RCT method do not suggest that it is inappropriate as a means of assessing the efficacy of alternative and complementary therapies; rather, their critiques centre on refinements of the RCT method (Bossuyt 2001; Thomas and Fitter 1997).
6. See also Drew and Davies (2001) and Rawsthorne et al. (1999).
7. See Critchley et al. (2000); Delaunay et al. (2000); Eisenberg et al. (1993); Eisenberg et al. cited in Bender (1999); Ernst (2000a, 1999, 1997, 1995a, 1995b, 1994); Ernst and

Barnes (1998); Feigen and Tiver (1986); Gottlieb (2001); Lade (2000); Odsberg et al. (2001); Stubberfield et al. (1999); and Yamashita et al. (2001).

8. See Critchley et al. (2000); Eisenberg et al. Cited in Bender (1999); Ernst (2000a, 1997, 1995a); and Odsberg et al. (2001); and Yamashita et al. (2001).

9. See also paragraph 7.27 of the House of Lords (2000) *Select Committee Report on Alternative and Complementary Therapies.*

10. See Camara and Danao-Camara (1999); Ernst 1997; Fairfield et al. (1998); Kitai et al. (1998); Norheim and Fønnebø (2000); Oldendick et al. (2000); Owens et al. (1999); Resch et al. (1997); Stubberfield et al. (1999); Vincent and Furnham (1996); and Vincent et al. (1995).

11. See Dawson et al. (2000); Ernst (1997); Mitzdorf et al. (1999); and Zollman and Vickers (1999a, 1999b).

Appendix: The Therapies

Listed below are brief explanations of the alternative therapies and healing systems mentioned in this book. No consensus exists concerning how to define alternative or complementary health care (Low 2001a; Nahin and Straus 2001; Pawluch 1996). In addition, there are different schools of the same therapy and practitioners do not always agree about fundamentals of a therapeutic approach (Nahin and Straus 2001). Therefore, the following definitions are meant merely to acquaint readers with any therapies they may be unfamiliar with. In no way do I mean these descriptions to be understood as definitive, nor are they meant to necessarily represent what the people who participated in this research believe about any of these forms of health care. Consequently, I have selected definitions randomly from scholarly literature, popular sources, and advertising pamphlets. In addition, and in keeping with one of the primary aims of this research—highlighting the views of the lay user of alternative therapies—wherever possible I use quotations from informant interviews.

ACUPRESSURE

Acupressure is very similar to acupuncture except that the practitioner's hands, rather than needles, are used to balance the energy[1] which flows along the meridians of the body (Fulder 1996).

ACUPUNCTURE

Acupuncture has been used as a traditional method of healing in China for the last five thousand years. The intent is to "bring about a balance between positive and negative (*yin-yang*) ... energy [which] travels throughout the body by means of pathways called meridians" (Crockett 1996). It involves the insertion of thin needles into the body at precise points along these meridians; these needles are sometimes jiggled to increase the healing effect (Crockett 1996). While some techniques of Western acupuncture are similar to traditional Chinese acupuncture, the healing paradigm it is based on is consistent with a biomedical understanding of health, illness, and the body rather than with the health and healing ideology that underpins traditional Chinese medicine. For instance, medical research has "linked acupuncture points to certain types of nerve endings and demonstrated that needling causes the release of natural pain killers" (Vickers 1993:120).

AROMATHERAPY

According to Gaylord (1999:42), "Aromatherapy is a term coined in 1937 ... by the French chemist René Maurice Gattefoss." Aromatherapy involves smelling different essences and oils, where each oil "has its own property and is particularly effective for certain conditions" (Parkinson's Disease Society 1998/99:10–11). Most often the oils are applied during massage: "[a] method allow[ing] the oils both to be inhaled and be absorbed into ... the skin, as well as bringing the traditional benefits of massage" (Parkinson's Disease Society 1998/99:10).

ASTROLOGICAL HEALING

Astrological healing is a therapeutic approach that uses a person's astrological sign as a reference point in diagnosis and treatment of ill health (field notes). Astrological healing is based on the doctrine of the "'zodiacal man' [where] each of the twelve signs ... of the zodiac govern a different part of the ... body," and on the idea that particular "'planetary configurations'" can make the individual vulnerable to disease (*Alternative health dictionary* 2003).

BAGUA

Bagua is a healing form of martial arts "based in part on the ... *I Ching*" (*Body, mind, harmony* 2003). It involves "Taoist circular walking practice ... developed by Dong Hai-Chuan, ... during the mid 1800s" (*Alternative health dictionary* 2003). Randal, one of the people I spoke with, offers this perspective:

I met a person who was doing this kind called *Bagua Chi Gun*. She was using it to control her epilepsy, and her epileptic seizures, and some other stuff within her life. Since she had started it, and within the first six months, she had had two attacks. And for the year and a half after that she had no attacks, where she used to have five to seven attacks a day. I said: 'This is a healing form!' And she was telling me about someone else in her class who was using it to control their blood sugar level and I thought wow! neat! And it was very gentle. It is based upon circular stuff, people travel in circles, people's spirit.

CHINESE HERBAL MEDICINE

There are four main categories of Chinese medicine: "Chinese herbalism, Chinese food cures, Chinese acupuncture, and Chinese manipulative therapies" (Lu 1991). They all rest on the assumption that "all things in the animate and inanimate world are ... dynamic interactions" (Porkert and Ullmann 1988:73). In terms of health, Chinese medicine sees the individual as "a constellation of energy rather than a physical body which is inhabited by a soul or spirit" (Porkert and Ullmann 1988:84). Disease is conceptualized as a disturbance in the harmonious balance of energy that constitutes the human being (Porkert and Ullmann 1988). Among the causes of disease are: "external factors (wind, cold, summer heat, dampness, dryness, and fire), internal factors (joy, anger, worry, thought, sadness, fear, and shock), and two other causes which are neither internal nor external, fatigue and foods" (Lu 1991:31). Herbal decoctions[2] in conjunction with other modalities within Chinese medicine, serve to restore harmony or health to the individual (Porkert and Ullmann 1988).

CHIROPRACTIC

Chiropractic developed out of Osteopathy, which views "disease as primarily a result of problems with the skeletal and muscular systems resulting in obstruction of circulatory system" (Northcott 1994:494). Specifically, chiropractic therapy is concerned with manipulation of the spine. Many chiropractors believe that disease is a result of the misalignment of the spine and that readjustment serves to bring the person back to health and well-being (Northcott 1994). According to the Ontario Chiropractic Association brochure *Facts About Chiropractic:*

> Chiropractic is the science which concerns itself with the relationship between structure, primarily the spine, and function, primarily the nervous system, of the human body as the relationship may affect the restoration and preservation of health. (Clarke 1996:349)

While chiropractors generally concentrate on the spine, many also use nutrition, homeopathic remedies, and lifestyle counselling amongst their therapeutic modalities. This is because until very recently most chiropractors in Canada held dual classifications as naturopaths (Clarke 1996).

CHRISTIAN SCIENCE MEDICINE

Christian Science Medicine is a spiritual healing system that rejects allopathic medicine. According to Mary Baker Eddy (1934:109–123), founder of the Christian Science religion: "The term Christian Science ... designate[s] the scientific system of divine healing [and] reveals incontrovertibly that mind is All-in-all, that the only realities are the divine Mind and idea." The Christian Science approach to healing can be summed up in the principles "God is All-in-all; God is good God is Mind; God, Spirit, being all, nothing is matter; Life, God, omnipotent good, deny death, evil, sin, disease" (Eddy 1934:113). In other words, illness and disease are seen as errors of the mind. Only through prayer and divine intervention can they be corrected, returning the person to health. According to Randal,

> Christian Science was a good experience for me. And there was always testimony of healing and how you saw it interact in your life. You sort of shared in conducting that experience and where you found quotes within the bible ... that would help you along that turning point. I heard stories of people getting over cancer, people who were born blind seeing without glasses.

CREATIVE VISUALIZATION

Creative visualization was popularized by Shakti Gawain in the late 1970s. As a therapeutic medium, healing is accomplished by using the power of the mind to effect the elimination of illness or disease. For example, to cure oneself of cancer using this approach, one concretely imagines the destruction of the tumour or cancerous cells "regularly until it becomes reality," endowing the visualization with positive energy throughout the process of healing (*Alternative health dictionary* 2003).

CRYSTAL HEALING

Crystal healing is based on the notion that certain stones can be used as conduits for healing energy. Each stone has different healing properties (Thompson 1989). One of the participants in this research, Jane, offered to give me a crystal healing session. She asked me to sit down and hold my feet up slightly while she held two crystals at the soles of my feet. She told me that the crystals were creating a circuit of positive energy that would course through my body. Positive energy would enter my body through my right foot, travel up and around my body, and push negative energy out through the bottom of my left foot. She also diagnosed as she treated, telling me I had had an injury to my shoulder some years ago. At the end of the session she pronounced me "pretty okay" (field notes).

EAR CANDLING

Purported to have its "origin in ancient Egyptian, Chinese, and North American Indian cultures," ear candling is one of a number of ways to remove toxins from the body (Natural Health Centre 1997). Specifically, it is a method of removing wax and other debris from the ear canal. This therapy is meant to improve hearing, vision, taste, smell, balance, and/or treat ear infections, sinus problems, dizziness, itching, and headaches (Bauer 1997).

Having had periodic problems with pain in my ears, I was curious to experiment with ear candling. I asked one informant, Marie, if she would give me a treatment. She briefly explained how ear candles are made and used. A hollow candle, wider at one end than the other, is made by wrapping cotton tape around a narrow cylinder, such as a pencil, which is then dipped in bee's wax (field notes). The narrower end of the candle is placed in the client's ear and "the opposite end of the candle is lit ... creat[ing] a warm vacuum effect [that] dislodges wax and other debris and pulls it into the unburnt section of the candle" (Bauer 1997). In Marie's words:

> People with ear problems, they've gone through procedures of having their ears syringed and it's rather uncomfortable. Ear candling is much

gentler. A very old ancient way of cleaning the debris out of the ear and I usually do it twice, a week apart.

During the treatment I lay on my side while the candle was placed in my ear and lit. As the candle burned down I heard a rushing sound that wasn't unpleasant. When both ears had been treated Marie cut open one of the burnt candles to show me the wax and dirt that had been removed from my ear.

FASTING

Fasting is a form of detoxification therapy, a method of healing that involves purging the body of impurities, toxins, and waste. The theory is that this prevents illness and disease and maintains the body's ability to heal itself (Haas 1981). Fasting involves refraining from eating solid food and drinking only water, clear liquids, and/or fruit juices for a period of time in order to rid the body of its build up of toxins and waste. Scott, the one person who took part in this study who mentioned experiences with fasting, had mixed feelings about it as a method of healing. Initially he found that fasting made him feel better. In his words:

> I did a seven-day juice fast. There's this idea that when you are fasting and giving your body a break you can actually get more energy. I wanted to see what that was like and see if it was a way of getting more in touch with my body. It actually worked. I became aware of how my body gets hungry and then the hunger would just go away and it would come at regular times. Because I was just focussing on my hunger and focussing on my body it brought me back into my body. The other thing that was happening was there was the process of detoxification, particularly around excreting stuff. At one point during this fast I just got this incredible bunch of energy, for like twenty-four hours.

However, he then told me that he began to notice that friends who were fasting or on restricted diets appeared unhappy and sickly. This made him question the long-term efficacy of healing through fasting and concluded that healing lies in listening to your body rather than adhering rigidly to any particular regime. He put it this way:

> You end up with people who are radical vegans and macrobiotics who

are extremely resentful of the world because they're so miserable. That just changed everything for me. I stopped being a vegetarian, I stopped worrying about my diet, I started to eat what I want and ever since then that's been my approach to healing in terms of diet and physical things. I just listen to my body as much as I can. There have been times that I've craved fasting or I just haven't felt like eating so I don't eat.

FELDENKRAIS METHOD

According to the Holistic Centre Hamilton (1993:24), the Feldenkrais method "is a powerful way to improve the ease, grace, and comfort of our movements." Practitioners use "gentle meditative movements" to help the client become more aware of "habitual ways of moving" which are detrimental to their health and well-being (Holistic Centre Hamilton 1993:24). Roger, another participant in this study, sees potential for this method of healing to go beyond the purely physical. In his words: "It's work that's used with athletes and dancers to improve neuromuscular organization, the ease and grace of movement, that sort of thing. But then it also has ... [bearing on] education and psychotherapy."

HERBAL MEDICINE

According to Hoffmann (1988:7), "Herbalism is practised holistically." While drugs made from plants have been used in allopathic medicine since its beginnings, herbalists argue that isolating the active ingredient from an herb or plant is reductionist and decreases the healing potential of the remedy. Like homeopathy and naturopathy, herbalism rests on the assumption of self-healing. Hoffman (1988:19) writes: "The person who is 'ill' is in fact the healer. Aid can be sought from 'experts'... but ... healing comes from within, from truly embracing the life that flows within us. Herbs will aid in this process, but healing is inherent in being alive." The aid in question here is decoctions of various herbs and plants.

HOMEOPATHY

Homeopathy was developed "in the early 1800s by Samuel Hahnemann, a German physician" (Northcott 1994:493). It is a system of healing based on the "law of similarities" or the principle of like cures like (Craig 1988).

For example, if someone has a fever, rather than providing a remedy to reduce temperature, a homeopath would prescribe a minute dose of something that elevates temperature. This in turn stimulates the body's ability to heal itself. Homeopathic remedies most often come in the form of tinctures, granules, or tablets that have either an alcohol or lactose base. Homeopathic remedies are generally made up of "vegetable, animal, or mineral sources" (Craig 1988). These substances are diluted over and over, up to a million trillion trillion times, until imperceptible traces of them remain. The remedy is further "potentized by vigorous shaking at each step of the reduction or dilution" (Craig 1988).

HYPNOTHERAPY

According to Fulder (1996:xxii), hypnotherapy refers to "the use of hypnotic suggestion" to treat disease and psycho-social problems.

IRIDOLOGY

Often used by naturopaths, iridology is a diagnostic technique involving examination of the iris, the membrane behind the cornea of the eye (Fulder 1996).

MASSAGE

According to Vickers (1993:86), massage is "the common root of all touch therapies." Therapeutic massage is a form of body work[3] involving manipulation of the soft tissue and is said to "relieve pain, headaches, and tension-related syndromes; promote relaxation, alleviate swelling, correct poor posture, and improve circulation" (Gaylord 1999:39).

MEDITATION

In meditation, health is engendered through the use of relaxation techniques and focussed breathing which clear the mind and promote both physical and spiritual well-being (Fulder 1996).

MIDWIFERY

Midwifery involves a holistic and non-invasive approach to childbirth where the midwife avoids the use of medical technology and does not "disempower the parents ... [by] taking control of the birthing process" (Northcott 2002:466). According to Laura, "I wanted to deliver my baby and feel like I was in control of what was happening."

NATUROPATHY

Naturopathy is based on a belief "that health and illness are both natural components of a total human being—spirit, body, and mind" (Clarke 1996:351), and that people have the ability to heal themselves. Sickness is conceived of as a signal from the body that the person is in a "healing crisis" and therapy focuses on "stimulating the individuals' vital healing force" (Clarke 1996:352). Naturopaths stress "natural, drugless healing" (Northcott 1994:494) and make use of a number of different therapies, including homeopathic remedies, nutrition, herbal remedies, massage, yoga, and lifestyle modification.

PSYCHIC HEALING

Psychic healing is a metaphysical form of therapy that incorporates clairvoyant diagnosis and the treatment of ill health through "the channelling of 'psychic energy' ... through the 'healer'" to the person (*Alternative health dictionary* 2003).

REFLEXOLOGY

Foot reflexology is a system of diagnosis and healing that "recognizes the feet to be important indicators of the health/disease of the entire body" (Dychtwald 1986:60). For example, Hanna told me that

> Reflexology's probably similar to acupressure where it's stimulating the reflex pads in the head, hands, and feet that correspond to all the parts of the body. There's about seventy-two thousand nerve endings in your feet and all the body has to function through those nerves.

If an organ is unhealthy, the point on the foot corresponding to it will be "very sensitive to touch" and the organ in question can be healed through manipulation and massage of the relevant pressure point (Dychtwald

1986:60). For instance, in telling me about foot reflexology, Lorraine describes her experience of a treatment given to her by her cousin. In her words: "My cousin has gone into reflexology. She can work on your feet and honestly she'll hit spots and oh are they sore! Because every place in our body ends up in our feet. So she'll work that spot, she'll work my toes and I'll feel my sinuses draining."

REIKI

Reiki is thought to be based on an ancient Tibetan healing system that was revived by Dr. Mikao Usui in Japan in the mid-1800s (Brophy 1995). It is described as a "non-invasive drugless hands-off technique to assist you in achieving balance in the body/mind/spirit complex" (Brophy 1995) and "on your journey of physical/mental/emotional healing and spiritual growth" (Price 1997). In passing their hands close to and sometimes touching the body of the client, practitioners can transmit healing energy to the person (Fryns 1995). The practitioner is merely the medium: it is the person who heals himself or herself. According to Marie, *reiki* is

> very ancient Tibetan healing and it's channelling the universal energy through our hands to you. It's up to you. I channel the energy to you. I provide a safe environment full of love and light and a safe neutral place for you to do whatever you need to do [to heal].

THE RESULTS SYSTEM

The results system is a program of healing that incorporates elements of therapeutic touch, energy work, nutrition, detoxification therapy, metaphysical healing, and creative visualization as healing techniques. According to Natalie, "The results system is a system to heal your mind, body, and spirit all at once. And within four or five sessions a person can be healed by conversation, and by healing of the hand, and by their belief system." When Natalie refers to healing by their belief system, she means by using creative visualization and positive affirmations to replace negative thought patterns (Achterberg 1985). The healing process involves determining if there are blocks impeding the flow of energy within the person. In Natalie's words: "If the *chakras*[4] are blocked for any reason, due to stress, illness, disease, these have to be opened before you can possibly help this person." Natalie went on to describe how blocked *chakras* are detected and corrected:

> So each time you do this you can check with their fingers, baby finger and thumb touched together, whether that *chakra* is really open or not. If the fingers fly open as you pull your client's fingers apart then you know that *chakra* needs to be opened. Once you open the *chakra*, then you come back and touch that part of the *chakra* with your hand just gently and then do the fingers of the client and see if they're still open. If they stay tight you know you've got it open.

Once the *chakras* are opened healing with therapeutic touch can begin. In Natalie's words: "Once those are all cleared you can go forth and try to heal this person with your hands." The results system also incorporates the notion of harnessing universal energy to help people heal themselves. Natalie told me that the results system is based on the metaphysical belief that a higher power is guiding the healing. She said: "There's somebody directing this. It could be spirits, it could be angels, but above all that there is one person, like a god."

THERAPEUTIC TOUCH

Therapeutic touch, also referred to as healing touch, involves the transfer of energy from the practitioner to the client. By moving his or her hands close to, or lightly touching, the client's body, the practitioner enables the person to heal (field notes). According to Natalie:

> You put your hands above their head, about two, three inches away from them and you hold them there and then you go over the entire body. And you can feel different spots in their body where they have a problem. It's like a vibration comes to your hand. Heat sensation or a prickling of the fingers.

VITAMIN THERAPY

Vitamin therapy is based on the belief that imbalances of nutrients in the body create ill health and that certain "vitamins ... [are] a potent means of influencing body chemistry and thus disease processes" (Fulder 1996:250). In the mid-1960s, Norman Cousins popularized the use of megadoses of vitamin C as a therapeutic approach.

YOGA

Yoga is a system of balancing bodily energy through stretching the body, regulating breathing, and putting the body into specific postures (Kabat-Zin 1993). According to Hanna,

> Yoga, to our knowledge, is at least five thousand years old. The word yoga means union. It's the union between body, mind, and spirit and physically it works on the endocrine system. When the endocrine system's not functioning properly then the hormones aren't secreting into the body, there's an imbalance and that's where ill health comes from. So the postures are designed to squeeze and release, increase blood flow and hormonal supply into the system to help the body get balanced, and then the body can help itself.

Healing through yoga means building up and controlling bodily energy or life force. In Hanna's words: "It's energy and the more you do your yoga breathing, the more *prana* you get in there. And you build it and build it until it builds up a resistance against illnesses and diseases. We call it *pranayama* which means life force control."

NOTES

1. What is common to many therapies involving energy as a therapeutic medium is that they rest on the notion that every living thing is imbued with energy or a life force and that total well-being depends on the balanced flow of this energy (Blate 1982). In addition, spiritual energy, universal energy, and/or the energy within the natural world can be harnessed to heal (Blate 1982).
2. "A liquor containing the concentrated essence of a substance, produced as a result of heating... used in medicinal and herbal preparations" (Pearsall 1999:372).
3. Body work is based in part on the belief that disease is caused by the build up of physical and emotional trauma that is stored in the musculature of the body. By manipulating the musculature, tension and "the chronically held traumas of a lifetime are removed," allowing a return to health and well-being (Dychtwald, 1986:12).
4. There are seven *chakras*, or spiritual centres, along the body which govern different aspects of mind, body, and spirit (Dychtwald 1986). For instance, the "root *chakra* [is] located at the base of the spine [and] relates to ... primitive energy and basic survival needs" (Dychtwald 1986:87)

References

Aakster, C. W. (1986). Concepts in alternative medicine. *Social Science and Medicine,* 22(2):265–273.

Achilles, R. (2001). Defining complementary and alternative health care. In Health Canada, *Perspectives on complementary and alternative health care,* pp. I.11–15.

Achilles, R., Adelson, N., Antze, P., and Biggs, C. L. (1999). *Complementary and alternative health practices and therapies—A Canadian overview.* Toronto: York University Centre for Health Studies.

Achterberg, J. (1985). *Imagery in healing.* Boston: New Science Library, Shambhala Publications Limited.

Alternative Medicine Dictionary. (2003). Publication on the Internet, viewed 2 September, 2003, http://www.canoe.ca/altmeddictionary/a.html

Angus Reid Group Inc. (1998). Use and Danger of Alternative Medicines and practice: Parts I and II. Consumer poll conducted by CTV/Angus Reid, August 1997.

Anyinam, C. (1990). Alternative medicine in Western countries: An agenda for medical geography. *The Canadian Geographer,* 34(1):69–76.

Archer, M. S. (1988). *Culture and agency: The place of culture in social theory.* Cambridge: Cambridge University Press.

Armstrong, P. and Armstrong, H. (1996). *Wasting away: The undermining of Canadian health care.* Toronto: Oxford University Press.

Babbie, E. (1986). *The practice of social research.* California: Wadsworth Publishing Company.

Bakx, K. (1991). The 'eclipse' of folk medicine in western society. *Sociology of Health and Illness,* 13(1):20–38.

Balon, J. W., Best, A., Kelner, M., La Valley, J. W., Rickhi, B., Savas, D., Soucy-Hirtle, F., Thorne, S., Verspoor, R., Shearer, R., and Simpson, J. E. (2001a). Towards an integrative health system. In Health Canada, *Perspectives on complementary and alternative health care,* pp. IV.45–52.

Balon, J. W., Best, A., Kelner, M., La Valley, J. W., Rickhi, B., Savas, D., Soucy-Hirtle, F., Thorne, S., Verspoor, R., Shearer, R., and Simpson, J. E. (2001b). The need for guidelines: Ethical issues in the use of complementary and alternatvie health care in Canada today. In Health Canada, *Perspectives on complementary and alternative health care,* pp. III.41–44.

Barton, S. (2000). Which clinical studies provide the best evidence? *British Medical Journal,* 321:255–256.

Bauer, G. (1997). Bloom 'n' Gales Aromatherapy/Massage/Ear Candling [advertising flyer]. (Available from Gail Bauer 3487 Hwy. #6, Mount Hope, Ontario, L0R 1W0).

Becker, H. S. (1970a). *Sociological work: Method and substance*. Chicago: Aldine.

Becker, H. S. (1970b). Problems of inference and proof in participant observation. In W. J. Filstead (Ed.), *Qualitative methodology: Firsthand involvement with the social world*, pp. 189–201. Chicago: Markham Publishing Company.

Becker, H. S. (1966). Introduction. In C. Shaw, *The jack-roller: A delinquent boy's own story*, pp. v–xix. Chicago: University of Chicago Press.

Becker, H. S. and Strauss, A. L. (1956). Careers, personality, and adult socialization. *American Journal of Sociology*, 62:253–263.

Bender, K. (1999). Scientific assessment of alternative medicine. *Psychiatric Times*, 16(2):41–42.

Berger, P. (1963). *Invitation to sociology: A humanistic perspective*. Garden City, New York: Anchor Books, Doubleday and Company Ltd.

Berliner, H. S. and Salmon, J. W. (1979a). The new realities of health policy and influences of holistic medicine. *C/O: Journal of Alternative Human Services*, 5(2):13–16.

Berliner, H. S. and Salmon, J. W. (1979b). The holistic health movement and scientific medicine: the naked and the dead. *Socialist Review*, 9(1):31–52.

Birch, S. (1997). Issues to consider in determining an adequate treatment in a clinical trial of acupuncture. *Complementary Therapies in Medicine*, 5:8–12.

Blais, R. (2000). Changes in characteristics of CAM users over time. In M. Kelner, B. Wellman, B. Pescosolido, and M. Saks (Eds.), *Complementary and alternative medicine: Challenge and change*, pp. 115–129. The Netherlands: Harwood Academic Publishers.

Blate, M. (1982). *How to heal yourself using hand acupressure (hand reflexology)*. Davie, Florida: Falkynor Books.

Blumer, H. (1969). *Symbolic interactionism: Perspective and method*. New Jersey: Prentice Hall Inc.

Body, mind, harmony. (2003). Publication on the Internet, viewed 2 September, 2003, http:www.bodymindharmony.com/bagua.html

Boon, H. (1998). The making of a naturopathic practitioner: The education of alternative practitioners. *Health and Canadian Society*, 3(1 and 2):5–41.

Boon, H., Brown, J. B., Gavin, A., Kennard, M. A., Stewart, M. (1999). Breast cancer survivors' perceptions of complementary/alternative medicine: making the decision to use or not use. *Qualitative Health Research*, 9(5):639–653.

Bossuyt, P. M. M. (2001). Better standards for better reporting of RCTs. *British Medical Journal*, 322:1317–1318

Bourgeault, I. (2000). Delivering the 'new' Canadian midwifery: The impact on midwifery of integration into the Ontario health care system. *Sociology of Health and Illness*, 22(2):172–96.

Bourgeault, I. and Fynes, M. (1997). Integrating lay and nurse-midwifery into the U. S. and Canadian health care systems. *Social Science and Medicine*, 44(7):1051–63.

Boutin, P. D., Buchwald, D., Robinson, L. and Collier, A. C. (2000). Use of and attitudes about alternative and complementary therapies among outpatients and physicians at a municipal hospital. *Journal of Alternative and Complementary Medicine*, 6(4):335–343.

Brophy, M. (1995). *Reiki: The Usui System of Natural Healing* [advertising pamphlet]. (Marguerite Brophy, Hamilton, Ontario).

Bury, M. (1991). The sociology of chronic illness: A review of research and prospects. *Sociology of Health and Illness*, 13(4):451–468.

Bury, M. (1982). Chronic illness as biographic disruption. *Sociology of Health and Illness*, 4(2):167–182.

Cain, R., Pawluch, D. Gillet, J. (1999). *Practitioner perspectives on complementary therapy use among people living with HIV*. McMaster University/Health Canada.

Calmels, P. (1999). A scientific perspective on developing acupuncture as a complementary medicine. *Disability and Rehabilitation*, 21(3):129–130.

Camara, K. and Danao-Camara, T. (1999). Awareness of, use, and perception of efficacy of alternative therapies by patients with inflammatory arthropathies. *Hawaii Medical Journal*, 58:329–332

Campion, E. W. (1993). Why unconventional medicine? *New England Journal of Medicine*, 318(4):282–283.

Canada Health Monitor. (1993). *Survey # 9*. Price Waterhouse, Toronto, Ontario, CT: Earl Berger.

Canadian Institute for Health Information. (2002). *Health care in Canada*. Ottawa: Statistics Canada.

CMAJ (1991). One in five Canadians is using alternative therapies, survey finds. *Canadian Medical Association Journal*, 144(4):469.

Cant, S. L. and Calnan, M. (1991). On the margins of the medical marketplace? An exploratory study of alternative practitioners' perspectives. *Sociology of Health and Illness*, 13(1):39–57.

Cant, S. L. and Sharma, U. (1995). *Professionalisation in complementary medicine*. UK: Economic and Social Research Council Report.

Cassee, E. T. (1970). Deviant illness behaviour: Patients of mesmerists. *Social Science and Medicine*, 3:389–396.

Casey, J. and Picherack, F. (2001). The regulation of complementary and alternative health care practitioners: Policy considerations. In Health Canada, *Perspectives on complementary and alternative health care*, pp. VI. 63–86.

Charmaz, K. (1991). Fictional identities and turning points. In D. R. Maines (Ed.), *Social organization and social processes: Essays in honour of Anselm Strauss*, pp. 71–86. New York: Aldine de Gruyter.

Charmaz, K. (1987). Struggling for a self: Identity levels of the chronically ill. *Research in the Sociology of Health Care*, 6:283–321.

Charmaz, K. (1983). Loss of self: a fundamental form of suffering in the chronically ill. *Sociology of Health and Illness*, 5(2):168–195.

Chrisman, N. J. and Kleinman, A. (1983). Popular health care, social networks, and cultural meanings: The orientation of medical anthropology. In D. Mechanic (Ed.), *Handbook of health, health care, and the health professions*, pp. 569–590. New York: The Free Press, London: Collier-Macmillan Ltd.

Clarke, J. N. (1996). *Health, illness, and medicine in Canada*, second edition. Toronto: Oxford University Press.

Cobb, B. (1958). Why do people detour to quacks? In E. Jaco (Ed.), *Patients, physicians, and illness*, pp. 283–287. New York: The Free Press.

Coburn, D. (1997). State authority, medical dominance and trends in the regulation of the health professions: The Ontario case. In J. K. Crellin, R. R. Andersen, and J. T. H. Connor (Eds.), *Alternative health care in Canada*, pp. 92–109. Toronto: Canadian Scholars' Press Inc.

Coburn, D. and Biggs, L. (1987). Chiropractic: Legitimation or medicalization? In D. Coburn, C. D'Arcy, G. Torrance (Eds.), *Health and Canadian society: Sociological perspectives*, pp. 366–384. Richmond Hill, Ontario: Fitzhenry and Whiteside.

Cockerham, W. C. (1998). *Medical sociology*, seventh edition. New Jersey: Prentice Hall.

Cohen, A. (1985). *The symbolic construction of community*. London: Tavistock.

Connor, J. T. H. (1997). 'A sort of Felo-de Se:' Eclecticism, related medical sects, and their decline in Victorian Ontario. In J. K. Crellin, R. R. Andersen, and J. T. H. Connor (Eds.), *Alternative health care in Canada*, pp. 59–83. Toronto: Canadian Scholars' Press Inc.

Conrad, P. and Schneider, J. W. (1980). *Deviance and medicalization: From badness to sickness.* C. V. Mosby and Company.

Corbin, J. M. and Strauss, A. L. (1990). Grounded theory research: Procedures, canons, and evaluative criteria. *Qualitative Sociology,* 13(1):3–21.

Corbin, J. M. and Strauss, A. L. (1988). *Unending work and care: Managing chronic illness at home.* San Francisco: Jossey-Bass Publishers Inc.

Corbin, J. M. and Strauss, A. L. (1987). Accompaniments of chronic illness: Changes in body, self, biography, and biographical time. *Research in the Sociology of Health Care,* 6:249–281.

Coulter, I. D. (1985). The chiropractic patient: A social profile. *Journal of the Canadian Chiropractic Association,* 29(1):March, 25–28.

Coward, R. (1989). *The whole truth: The myth of alternative health.* London, Boston: Faber and Faber.

Craig, C. (1988). *Homeopathy: What it is, How it Works* [advertising pamphlet]. (Available from Standard Homeopathic Company, Box 61067, Los Angeles, CA, 90061, USA).

Crawford, R. (1984). A cultural account of 'health': Control, release, and the social body. In J. B. McKinlay (Ed.), *Issues in the political economy of health care,* pp. 60–93. New York: Tavistock.

Creedon, J. (1998). God with a million faces. Designer gold: In a mix-and-match world, why not create your own religion? *Utne Reader,* (88):July/August.

Crellin, J. K., Andersen, R. R., and Connor, J. T. H. (1997). *Alternative health care in Canada,* Toronto: Canadian Scholars' Press Inc.

Critchley, J. A. J. H., Zhang, Y., Suthisisang, C. C., Chan, T. Y. K., and Tomlinson, B. (2000). Alternative therapies and medical science: designing clinical trials of alternative/complementary medicines—Is evidence-based traditional Chinese medicine attainable? *Journal of Clinical Pharmacology,* 40:462–467.

Crockett, S. F. (1996). *Acupuncture* [advertising pamphlet]. (Available from Sean F. Crockett, Ambience Hair design, 13 Augusta Street, Hamilton, Ontario).

Crosby, D. (1999). Complementary care is rising in the health service on a tide of half truths. *NHS Magazine,* Autumn.

Csordas, T. J. (1983). The rhetoric of transformation in ritual healing. *Culture, Medicine and Psychiatry,* 7(4):333–375.

Dawson, M. T., Gifford, S., and Amezquita, R. (2000). Donde hay doctor?: folk and cosmopolitan medicine for sexual health among Chilean women living in Australia. *Culture, Health and Sexuality,* 2(1):51–68.

Davis, F. (1961). Deviance disavowal: The management of strained interaction by the visibly handicapped. *Social Problems* 9:120–140.

de Bruyn, T. (2001). Taking stock: policy issues associated with complementary and alternative health care. In Health Canada, *Perspectives on complementary and alternative health care,* pp. II.17–39.

Delaunay, P. (2000). Homeopathy may not be effective in preventing malaria. [Letter to the Editor]. *British Medical Journal,* 321:1288.

Deierlein, K. (1994). Ideology and holistic alternatives. In W. Kornblum and C. D. Smith (Eds.), *The healing experience: Readings on the social context of health care,* pp. 177–187. New Jersey: Prentice Hall.

Donnelly, W. J., Spykerboer, J. E., and Thong, Y. H. (1985). Are patients who use alternative medicine dissatisfied with orthodox medicine? *The Medical Journal of Australia,* 142:539–541.

Douglas, J. D. (1976). *Investigative social research: Individual and team research.* Beverley Hills: Sage Publications.

Drew, S. and Davies, E. (2001). Effectiveness of Ginko biloba in treating tinnitus: double blind, placebo controlled trial. *British Medical Journal*, 322:1–6.

Dunfield, J. F. (1996). Consumer perceptions of health care quality and the utilization of non-conventional therapy. *Social Science and Medicine*, 43(2):149–161.

Dychtwald, K. (1986). *Bodymind*. Los Angeles: Jeremy P. Tarcher Inc. Distributed by St. Martin's Press.

Easthope, G. (1993). The response of orthodox medicine to the challenge of alternative medicine in Australia. *Australian and New Zealand Journal of Sociology*, 29(3):289–301.

Eddy, M. B. (1934). *Science and health with key to the scriptures*. Boston: The First Church of Christ, Scientist.

Eisenberg, D. M., Davis, R. B., Ettner, S. L. Appel, S., Wilkey, S., Van Rompay, M., and Kessler, R. C. (1998). Trends in alternative medicine use in the United States, 1990–97: Results of a follow-up national survey. *Journal of the American Medical Association*, 280(18):1569–1575.

Eisenberg, D. M., Kessler, R. C., Foster, C., Norlock. F. E., Clakins, D. R., Delbanco, T. L. (1993). Unconventional medicine in the United States: Prevalence, costs and patterns of use. *The New England Journal of Medicine*, 328(4):246–52.

Ernst, E. (2000a). Herbal medicines: Where is the evidence? *British Medical Journal*, 321:395–396.

Ernst, E. (2000b). The role of complementary and alternative medicine. *British Medical Journal*, 321:1133–1135.

Ernst, E. (1999). Evidence-based complementary medicine: A contradiction in terms? *Annals of the Rheumatic Diseases*, 58:69–70.

Ernst, E. (1997). Evidence-based complementary medicine. *Complementary Therapies in Nursing and Midwifery*, 3:42–45.

Ernst, E. (1995a). The risk of acupuncture. *International Journal of Risk and Safety in Medicine*, 6:179–186.

Ernst, E. (1995b). The safety of homeopathy. *British Homeopathy Journal*, 84:193–194.

Ernst, E. (1994). Cervical manipulation: Is it really safe? *International Journal of Risk and Safety in Medicine*, 6:145–149.

Ernst, E. and Barnes, J. (1998). Methodological approaches to investigating the safety of complementary medicine. *Complementary Therapies in Medicine*, 6:115–121.

Ernst, E. and Fugh-Berman, A. (1999). Complementary/alternative medicine—A critical review of acupuncture, homeopathy, and chiropractic. Paper presented at the Primary Care Groups and Complementary Medicine: Breaking the Boundaries conference. Department of Complementary Medicine, University of Exeter, Exeter, UK.

Eskinazi, D. P. (1998). Factors that shape alternative medicine. *Journal of the American Medical Association*, 280(18):1621–1623.

Evans, D. M. (1993). Three battles to watch in the 1990's. *Journal of the American Medical Association*, 270:520–526.

Fairfield, K. M., Eisenberg, D. M., Davis, R. B., Libman, H., and Phillips, R. S. (1998). Patterns of use, expenditures, and perceived efficacy of complementary and alternative therapies in HIV-infected patients. *Archives of Internal Medicine*, 150(Nov):2257–2264.

Feigen, M. and K. Tiver. (1986). The impact of alternative medicine on cancer patients. *Cancer Forum*, 10:15–19.

Fitter, M. J. and Thomas, K. J. (1997). Evaluating complementary therapies for use in the National Health Service: 'Horses for courses.' Part 1: The design challenge. *Complementary Therapies in Medicine*, 5: 90–93.

Fryns, T. (1995). *Reiki: The Usui System of Natural Healing* [advertising pamphlet]. (Available from Toni Fryns, Hamilton Holistic Centre, 500 James Street South, Hamilton, Ontario).

Fulder, S. J. (1996). *The handbook of alternative medicine*. Oxford: Oxford University Press.

Fulder, S. J. and Munro, R. E. (1985). Complementary medicine in the United Kingdom: Patients, practitioners, and consultants. *The Lancet*, 7 September, 542–45.

Furnham, A. (1994). Explaining health and illness: lay perceptions on current and future health, the causes of illness, and the nature of recovery. *Social Science and Medicine*, 39(5):715–725.

Furnham, A. and Beard, R. (1995). Health, just world beliefs, and coping style: Preferences in patients of complementary and orthodox medicine, *Social Science and Medicine*. 40(10):1425–32.

Furnham, A. and Bhagrath, R. (1993). A comparison of health beliefs and behaviours of orthodox and complementary medicine. *British Journal of Clinical Psychology*, 32:237–46.

Furnham, A. and Forey, J. (1994). The attitudes, behaviors, and beliefs of conventional vs. complementary (alternative) medicine. *Journal of Clinical Psychology*, 50(3):458–469.

Furnham, A. and Kirkcaldy, B. (1996). The health beliefs and behaviours of orthodox and complementary medicine clients. *British Journal of Clinical Psychiatry*, 35:49–61.

Furnham, A. and C. Smith. (1988). Choosing alternative medicine: A comparison of the beliefs of patients visiting a general practitioner and a homeopath. *Social Science and Medicine*, 26(7):685–689.

Furnham, A., Vincent, C., and Wood, R. (1995). The health beliefs and behaviours of three groups of complementary medicine and a general practice group. *Journal of Alternative and Complementary Medicine*, 1(4):347–359.

Gadsby, J. G., Franks, A. Jarvis, P., and Dewhurst, F. (1997). Acupuncture-like transcutaneous electrical nerve stimulation within palliative care: A pilot study. *Complementary Therapies in Medicine*, 5:13–18.

Gaylord, S. (1999). Alternative therapies and empowerment of older women. *Journal of Women and Aging*, 11(2/3):29–47

Gill, A. (2003). The new face of health care. *The Globe and Mail*, July 12, 2003:F6.

Gillett, G. (1994). Beyond the orthodox: Heresy in medicine and social science. *Social Science and Medicine*, 39(9):1125–1131.

Glaser, B. G. and Strauss, A. L. (1967). *The discovery of grounded theory: Strategies for qualitative research*. Chicago: Aldine Publishing.

Glik, D. C. (1990). Participation in spiritual healing, religiosity, and mental health. *Social Inquiry*, 60(2):58–176.

Glik, D. C. (1988). Symbolic, ritual and social dynamics of spiritual healing. *Social Science and Medicine*, 27(11):1197–1206.

Glik, D. C. and Kronenfeld, J. J. (1989). Well roles: An approach to reincorporate role theory into medical sociology. *Research into the Sociology of Health Care*, 8:289–309.

Goffman, E. (1963). *Stigma: Notes on the management of spoiled identity*. New Jersey: Prentice Hall Inc.

Goldstein, M. S., Jaffe, D. T., Sutherland, C., and Wilson, J. (1987). Holistic physicians: Implications for the study of the medical profession. *Journal of Health and Social Behaviour*, 28(June):103–119.

Gort, E. H. and Coburn, D. (1997). Naturopathy in Canada. In J. K. Crellin, R. R. Andersen, and J. T. H. Connor (Eds.), *Alternative health care in Canada*, pp. 143–171. Toronto: Canadian Scholars' Press Inc.

Gottlieb, S. (2001). No evidence that placebos have powerful clinical effects, study says. *British Medical Journal*, 322:1325.

Gottlieb, S. (2000). Patient dies after alternative remedy. *British Medical Journal*, 321:1491b.

Gray, R. E., Fitch, M., and Greenberg, M. (1998). Comparison of physician and patient perspectives on unconventional cancer therapies. *Psycho-Oncology*, 7:445–452.

Haas, E. M. (1981). *Staying healthy with the seasons*. Berkeley, California: Celestial Arts.

Hamilton, D. and Bechtel G. A. (1996). Research implications for alternative health therapies. *Nursing Forum*, 31(1):6–11.

Hare, M. L. (1993). The emergence of an urban U.S. Chinese medicine. *Medical Anthropology Quarterly*, 7(1):30–49.

Hart, A. (2001). Randomized control trials: The control group dilemma revisited. *Complementary Therapies in Medicine*, 9:40–44.

Haviland, D. (1992). The differing natures of alternative and complementary medicine. *International Journal of Alternative and Complementary Medicine;* 10: 27–28.

Health Canada. (2001). *Perspectives on complementary and alternative health care: A collection of papers prepared for Health Canada*. Ottawa: Health Canada Publications.

Hedley, R. A. (1992). Industrialization and the practice of medicine: Movement and countermovement. *International Journal of Comparative Sociology*, 33(3–4):208–214.

Heeney, H. (1995). *Life before Medicare: Canadian experiences*. The Stories Project, Ontario Coalition of Senior Citizens Organization.

Hoffmann, D. (1988). *The holistic healer*. Longmead, Shaftbury, Dorset: Element Books Ltd.

Holistic Centre, Hamilton (1993). *Calendar of Events and Classes* [Class schedule]. (Available from the Holistic Centre, 500 James Street North, Suite 200, Hamilton, Ontario, L8L 1J4).

House of Lords. (2000). *Complementary and Alternative Medicine, Select Committee on Science and Technology* [online]. URL: http://www.publications.parliment.uk. Accessed 12 April 2000.

Illich, I. (1975). *Medical nemesis: The expropriation of health*. Toronto: McClellan and Stewart.

Jingfeng, C. (1987). Toward a comprehensive evaluation of alternative medicine. *Social Science and Medicine*, 25(6):659–667.

Jobst, K. A. (2000). There are more things in medicine and science than are dreamt of in our paradigm, practice and policy! *The Journal of Alternative and Complementary Medicine*, 6(4):295–298.

Johnson, J. E. (1999). Older rural women and the use of complementary therapies. *Journal of Community Health Nursing*, 16(4):223–232.

Jones, L. (1987). Alternative Therapies: A report on an inquiry by the British Medical Association. *The Skeptical Inquirer*, 12(Fall):63–69.

Kabat-Zin, J. (1993). Meditation. In B. Moyers (Ed.), *Healing and the Mind*, pp. 115–143. New York: Doubleday.

Kacperek, L. (1997). Patients' views on the factors which would influence the use of aromatherapy massage out-patient service. *Complementary Therapies in Nursing and Midwifery*, 3:51–57.

Kelner, M. (2000). The therapeutic relationship under fire. In M. Kelner, B. Wellman, B. Pescosolido, and M. Saks (Eds.), *Complementary and alternative medicine: Challenge and change*, pp. 79–97. The Netherlands: Harwood Academic Publishers.

Kelner, M., Hall, O., and Coulter, I. (1986). *Chiropractors: Do they help?: A study of their education and practice*. Markham, Ontario: Fitzhenry and Whiteside.

Kelner, M. and Wellman, B. (2000). Introduction. In M. Kelner, B. Wellman, B. Pescosolido, and M. Saks (Eds.), *Complementary and alternative medicine: Challenge and change*, pp. 1–24. The Netherlands: Harwood Academic Publishers.

Kelner, M. and Wellman, B. (1997). Health care and consumer choice: Medical and alternative therapies. *Social Science and Medicine*, 45(2):203–212.

Kelner, M. Wellman, B., Pescosolido, B., and Saks, M. (2000). *Complementary and alternative medicine: Challenge and change*. The Netherlands: Harwood Academic Publishers.

Kirk, J. and Miller, M. L. (1986). *Reliability and validity in qualitative research*. Newbury Park: Sage Publications.

Kitai, E., Vinker, S., Sandiuk, A., Hornik, O., Zeltcher, C., and Gaver, A. (1998). Use of complementary and alternative medicine among primary care patients. *Family Practice*, 15(5): 411–414.

Knipschild, P., Kleijnen, J., and Reit, G. (1990). Belief in the efficacy of alternative medicine among general practitioners in the Netherlands. *Social Science and Medicine*, 31(5):625–626.

Kottow, M. H. (1992). Classical medicine v alternative medical practices. *Journal of Medical Ethics*, 18:18–22.

Kronenfeld, J. J. and Wasner, C. (1982). The use of unorthodox therapies and marginal practitioners. *Social Science and Medicine*, 16:1119–1125

Lade, H. (2000). Only one death from alternative cancer treatment. Publication on the Internet, viewed 16 December, 2003, http://www.bmj.com/eletters/321/7275/1491/b.

Latham, R. and Mathews, W., Eds. (1995). *The diary of Samuel Pepys 1663*. Los Angeles: Harper Collins Publishers.

Launsø, L. (2000). Use of alternative treatments in Denmark: Patterns of use and patients experience with treatment effects. *Alternative Therapies*, 6(1):102–107.

Leech, P. (1999). Complementary medicine, RSM. Paper presented at the conference: Primary Care Groups and Complementary Medicine: Breaking the Boundaries. Department of Complementary Medicine, University of Exeter, Exeter, UK.

Leibovici, L. (1999). Alternative (complementary) medicine: A cuckoo in the nest of empiricist reed warblers. *British Medical Journal*, 319:1629–1632.

Lemert, E. (1951). *Social pathology*. New York: McGraw Hill.

Lewith, G. T., Ernst, E., Mills, S., Fisher, P. Monckton, J., Reilly, D., Peters, D., and Thomas, K. (2000). Complementary medicine must be research led and evidence based. [Letter to the Editor]. *British Medical Journal*, 320:188.

Lindenmuth, G. F. and Lindenmuth, E. B. (2000). The efficacy of Echinacea compound herbal tea preparation on the severity and duration of upper respiratory and flu symptoms: A randomized, double-blind placebo controlled study. *Journal of Alternative and Complementary Medicine*, 6(4):327–334.

Lindsey, E. (1996). Health within illness: Experiences of chronically ill/disabled people. *Journal of Advanced Nursing*, 24(3):465–472.

Long, A. F., Mercer, G., and Hughes, K. (2000). Developing a tool to measure holistic practice: a missing dimension in outcomes measurement within complementary therapies. *Complementary Therapies in Medicine*, 8(1):26–31.

Low, J. (2004). Managing safety and risk: The experiences of people with Parkinson's disease who use alternative and complementary therapies. *Health: An Interdisciplinary Journal for the Study of Health, Illness and Medicine* (forthcoming).

Low, J. (2003). Lay assessments of the efficacy of alternative/complementary therapies: A challenge to medical and expert dominance? *Journal of Evidence-based Integrative Medicine*, 1(1):65–76.

Low, J. (2001a). Alternative, complementary, or concurrent health care? A critical analysis of the use of the concept of complementary therapy. *Complementary Therapies in Medicine*, 9(2):105–110.

Low, J. (2001b). *Lay perspectives on the efficacy of alternative and complementary therapies: The experiences of people living with Parkinson's disease*. Division of Health Studies, Faculty of Health and Community Studies, De Montfort University, Leicester, UK.

Low, J. (2000). Managing Stigma via retrospective reinterpretation: An analysis of individual-s' accounts of why they use alternative therapies. Paper presented at the British Sociological Association Medical Sociology Group and the European Society of Health and Medical Sociology Association Joint Conference. University of York, York, UK, September 14–17.

Lowenberg, J. S. (1992). *Caring and responsibility: The crossroads between holistic practice and traditional medicine.* Philadelphia: University of Pennsylvania Press.

Lu, H. C. (1991). *Legendary Chinese healing herbs.* New York: Sterling Publishing Company.

Lupton, D. (1997). Consumerism, reflexivity and the medical encounter. *Social Science and Medicine*, 45(3):373–381.

Maines, D. R. (1981). Recent developments in symbolic interaction. In G. P. Stone and Faberman, H. A. (Eds.), *Social psychology through symbolic interaction*, pp. 461–486. New York: Wiley.

Mason, F. (1993). *Overcoming barriers in the use of complementary therapies by persons living with HIV and AIDS.* Canadian AIDS Society.

McCracken, G. (1988). *The long interview.* Newbury Park: Sage Publications.

McGuire, M. B. (1988). *Ritual healing in suburban America.* London: Rutgers University Press.

McGuire, M. B. (1987). Ritual, symbolism and healing. *Social Compass*, 34(4):365–379.

McGuire, M. B. (1983). Words of power: Personal empowerment and healing. *Culture, Medicine and Psychiatry*, 7:221–240.

McGuire, M. B. and Kantor, D. J. (1987). Belief systems and illness experiences: The case of non-medical healing groups. *Research in the Sociology of Health Care*, 6:221–248.

Meade, T. W., Dyer, S., Browne, W. Townsend, J., and Frank, A. O. (1990). Low back pain of mechanical origin: Randomised comparison of chiropractic and hospital outpatient treatment. *British Medical Journal*, 300:1431–1437.

Mills, S. (2001). The House of Lords report on complementary medicine: A summary. *Complementary Therapies in Medicine*, 9:34–39.

Miller, M., Boyer, M. J., Butow, P. N., Gattellari, M., Dunn, S. M., and Childs, A. (1998). The use of unproven methods of treatment by cancer patients. *Support Care Cancer*, 6:337–347.

Miller, L. J. and Findlay, D. A. (1994). Through medical eyes: The medicalization of women's bodies and women's lives. In S. B. Bolaria and H. D. Dickinson (Eds.), *Health, illness and health care in Canada*, pp. 276–306. Canada: Harcourt Brace and Co. Ltd.

Mishler, E. G. (1989). Critical perspective on the biomedical model. In P. Brown (Ed.), *Perspectives in Medical Sociology*, pp. 153–166. Belmont, California: Wadsworth Publishing Company.

Mitzdorf, U., Beck, K., Horton-Hausknecht, J., Weidenhammer, W., Kindermann, A., Takács, Astor, G., and Melchart, D. (1999). Why do patients seek treatment in hospitals of complementary medicine? *Journal of Alternative and Complementary Medicine*, 5(5):463–473.

Moenkhoff, M., Baenziger, O., Fischer, J., and Fanconi, S. (1999). Parental attitude towards alternative medicine in the paediatric intensive care unit. *European Journal of Paediatrics*, 158:12–17.

Mohawk College, Hamilton, Ontario (2003a). [Course catalogue]. Publication on the Internet, viewed 10 June, 2003, http://www.mohawkc.on.ca/dept/cehs/index.html

Mohawk College, Hamilton, Ontario (2003b). [Course catalogue] Publication on the Internet, viewed 10 June, 2003, http://www.mohawkc.on.ca/dept/cehs/complementary.html

Mohawk College, Hamilton, Ontario (1998). *Mohawk College Continuing Education, Fall '98* (Available from Mohawk College, Fennell Campus, Fennell and West 5th, (905) 385–4295, Hamilton, Ontario, L8N 3T2).

Monson, N. (1995). Alternative medicine education at medical schools: Are they catching on? *Journal of Alternative and Complementary Therapies*, 1(3):168–71.

Montbriand, M. J. and Laing, G. P. (1991). Alternative health care as a control strategy. *Journal of Advanced Nursing*, 16:325–332.

Moore, J., Phipps, K., and Marcer, D. (1985). Why do people seek treatment by alternative medicine? *British Medical Journal*, 20:28–29.

Murphy, D. G. (2000). Developing research methodology in spiritual healing: Definitions, scope and limitations. [Letter to the Editor]. *Journal of Alternative and Complementary Medicine*, 6(4):299–302.

Murray, R. H. and Rubel, A. J. (1992). Physicians and healers—unwitting partners in health care. *New England Journal of Medicine*, 326(1):61–64.

Murray, J. and Shepherd, S. (1993). Alternative or additional medicine? An exploratory study in general practice. *Social Science and Medicine*, 37(8):983–988.

Nahin, R .L. and Straus, S. E. (2001). Research into complementary and alternative medicine: problems and potential. *British Medical Journal*, 322:161–164.

Natural Health Centre. (1997). [advertising flyer]. (Available from 80 Norfolk Street South, Simcoe, Ontario)

Norheim, A. J. and Fønnebø, V. (2000). A survey of acupuncture patients: Results from a questionnaire among a random sample in the general population in Norway. *Complementary Therapies in Medicine*, 8:187–192.

Northcott, H. C. (2002). Health care restructuring and alternative approaches to health and medicine. In S. B. Bolaria and H. D. Dickinson (Eds.), *Health, illness, and health care in Canada*, third edition, pp. 460–474. Canada: Nelson.

Northcott, H. C. (1994). Alternative health care in Canada. In S. B. Bolaria and H. D. Dickinson (Eds.), *Health, illness, and health care in Canada*, second edition, pp. 487–503. Canada: Harcourt Brace and Co. Ltd.

Northcott, H. C. and Bachynsky, J. A. (1993). Concurrent utilization of chiropractic, prescription medicine, nonprescription medicines, and alternative health care. *Social Science and Medicine*, 37(3):431–435.

O'Connor, B. B. (1995). *Healing traditions: Alternative medicine and the health professions*, Philadelphia: University of Pennsylvania Press.

Odsberg, A., Schill, U., and Haker, E. (2001). Acupuncture treatment: Side effects and complications reported by Swedish physiotherapists. *Complementary Therapies in Medicine*, 9:17–20.

Oldendick, R., Coker, A. L., Wieland, D., Raymond, J. I., Probst, J. C., Schell, B. J., and Stoskopf, C. H. (2000). Population based survey of complementary and alternative medicine usage, patient satisfaction, and physician involvement. *Southern Medical Journal*, 93(4):375–381.

Owens, J. E., Taylor, A. G., and Degood, D. (1999). Complementary and alternative medicine and psychologic factors: Toward an individual differences model of complementary and alternative medicine use and outcomes. *Journal of Alternative and Complementary Medicine*, 5(6):529–541.

Parkinson's Disease Society. (1998/99). Complementary therapies. Part 1: Aromatherapy. *The Parkinson*, Winter:10–11.

Pawluch, D. (1996). Reflections on the Sociological study of 'alternative' health care. Paper Presented at the Qualitative Research Conference, Studying Human Lived Experience: Symbolic Interaction and Ethnographic Research '96, McMaster University, Hamilton, Ontario.

Pawluch, D., Cain, R., and Gillet, J. (1998a). Lay constructions of HIV/AIDS and complementary therapy use. Paper Presented at the 14th World Congress of Sociology, International Sociological Association, Montréal, Québec.

Pawluch, D., Cain, R., and Gillet, J. (1998b). *Approaches to complementary therapies: Diverse perspectives among people with HIV/AIDS.* Hamilton, Ontario, McMaster University.

Pawluch, D., Cain, R., and Gillet, J. (1994). Ideology and alternative therapy use among people living with HIV/AIDS. *Health and Canadian Society,* 2(1):63–84.

Pearsall, J., ed. (1999). *Concise Oxford Dictionary, Tenth Edition.* Oxford: Oxford University Press.

Perlman, A., D. Eisenberg, and R. Panush. (1999). Talking with patients about alternative and complementary medicine. *Rheumatic Disease Clinics of North America,* 25:815–822.

Pescosolido, B. A. (1998). Beyond rational choice: The social dynamics of how people seek help. In W. C. Cockerham, M. Glasser, and L. S. Heuser (Eds.), *Readings in medical sociology,* pp. 208–223. Chicago: University of Chicago Press.

Phripp, R. (1991). Ecological illness and the quest for medical legitimation. Paper Presented at the Qualitative Analysis Conference 1991, Carlton University, Ottawa, Ontario.

Porkert, M. P. and Ullmann, C. (1988). *Chinese medicine: Its history, philosophy, and practice, and why it may one day dominate the medicine of the West.* New York: William Morrow and Company, Inc.

Price, C. (1997). *White Light Healing Service* [advertising pamphlet]. (Available from Charles Price, Cambridge, Ontario).

Pretorius, E. (1993). Alternative (complementary?) medicine in South Africa. *South African Journal of Sociology,* 24(1):13–17.

Prus, R. (1997). *Subcultural mosaics and intersubjective realities.* Albany: State of New York University Press.

Ramsay, C., Walker, M., and Alexander, J. (1999). *Alternative medicine in Canada: Use and public attitudes.* Fraser Institute, Report No. 21.

Rawsthorne, P., Shanahan, F., Cronin, N. C., Anton, P. A., Löfberg, Bohman, L., and Bernstein, C. N. (1999). An international survey of the use and attitudes regarding alternative medicine by patients with inflammatory bowel disease. *The American Journal of Gastroenterology,* 94(5):1298–1303.

Resch, K. I., Ernst, E., and Garrow, J. (2000). A randomized controlled study of reviewer bias against an unconventional therapy. *Journal of the Royal Society of Medicine,* 93:164–167.

Resch, K. I., Hill, S., and Ernst, E. (1997). Use of complementary therapies by individuals with 'Arthritis.' *Clinical Rheumatology,* 16(4):391–395.

Riley, J. N. (1980). Client choices among osteopaths and ordinary physicians in a Michigan community. *Social Science and Medicine,* 14b:111–120.

Saks, M. (1998). Medicine and complementary medicine: Challenge and change. In G. Scambler and P. Higgs (Eds.), *Modernity, medicine and health,* pp. 198–215. London: Routledge.

Saks, M. (1997a). East meets west: The emergence of an holistic tradition. In R. Porter (Ed.), *Medicine: A history of healing,* pp. 196–221. London: Routledge.

Saks, M. (1997b). Alternative therapies: Are they holistic? *Complementary Therapies in Nursing and Midwifery,* 3:4–8.

Saks, M. (1996). From quackery to complementary medicine. In S. Cant and U. Sharma (Eds.), *Complementary and Alternative Medicines,* pp. 27–43. London: Free Association Books.

Saks, M. (1995). *Professions and the public interest: Medical power, altruism and alternative medicine,* London: Routledge.

Schneirov, M. and Geczik, J. D. (1996). A diagnosis for our times: Alternative health's submerged networks and the transformation of identity. *The Sociological Quarterly,* 37(4):627–644.

Scott, M. and S. Lyman. (1981). Accounts. In G. Stone and H. Faberman (Eds.), *Social psychology through symbolic interaction,* pp. 343–361. New York: Wiley.

Sévigny, O., Quéniart, A., Lippman, A., Hess, S., and Chabot, P. (1990). *L'évaluation des soins holistiques. International Review of Community Development,* 24(64):104–116.

Shaffir, W. B. and Stebbins, R. A. (1991). Introduction. In W. B. Shaffir and R. A. Stebbins (Eds.), *Experiencing field work: An inside view of qualitative research,* pp. 1–24. Newbury Park: Sage Publications.

Sharma, U. (1993). Contextualizing alternative medicine: The exotic, the marginal and the perfectly mundane. *Anthropology Today,* 9(4):15–18.

Sharma, U. (1992). *Complementary medicine today: Practitioners and patients.* London and New York: Tavistock/Routledge.

Sharma, U. (1990). Using alternative therapies: Marginal medicine and central concerns. In P. Abbott and G. Payne (Eds.), *New directions in the sociology of medicine,* pp. 127–139. London: The Falmer Press.

Smith, R. (1991). Where is the wisdom ...? *British Medical Journal,* 303:798–799.

Stambolovic, V. (1996). Medical heresy—the view of a heretic. *Social Science and Medicine,* 43(5):601–604.

Strauss, A. L. and Corbin, J. (1990). *Basics of qualitative research: Grounded theory procedures and techniques.* Newbury Park: Sage Publications.

Stubberfield, T. G., Wray, J. A., and Parry, T. S. (1999). Utilization of alternative therapies in attention-deficit hyperactivity disorder. *Journal of Paediatric and Child Health,* 35:450–453.

Sykes, G. and D. Matza. (1957). Techniques of neutralization. *American Sociological Review,* 22:667–669.

Tataryn, D. and Verhoef, M. J. (2001). Combining conventional, complementary, and alternative health care: A vision of integration. In Health Canada, *Perspectives on complementary and alternative health care,* pp. VII.87–109.

Taylor, M. A., Reilly, D., Llewellyn-Jones, R. H., McSharry, C., and Aitchison, T. C. (2000). Randomised controlled trial of homeopathy versus placebo in perennial allergic rhinitis with overview of four trial series. *British Medical Journal,* 321:471–476.

Taylor, R. C. R. (1984). Alternative medicine and medical encounters in Britain and the United States. In J. W. Salmon (Ed.), *Alternative medicines: Popular and policy perspectives,* pp. 191–228. New York, London: Tavistock Publications.

Thomas, K. J., Carr, J., Westlake, L., and Williams, B. T. (1991). Use of non-orthodox and conventional health care in Great Britain. *British Medical Journal,* 302:207–210.

Thomas, K. J. and Fritter, M. J. (1997). Evaluating complementary therapies for use in the National Health Service: 'Horses for courses.' Part 2: Alternative research strategies. *Complementary Therapies in Medicine,* 5:94–98.

Thomas, K. J., Nicholl, J. P., and Coleman, P. (2001). Use and expenditure on complementary medicine in England: A population based survey. *Complementary Therapies in Medicine,* 9:2–11.

Thomas, W. I. and Thomas, D. S. (1970). Cited in G. P. Stone and H. A. Faberman (Eds.), *Social psychology through symbolic interaction,* p. 154. New York: Wiley.

Thompson, C. J. S. (1989). *Magic and healing: The history of magical healing practices from herb-lore and incantations to rings and precious stones.* New York: Bell Publishing Company.

Tonkin, R. (1987). Research into complementary medicine. *Complementary Medical Research,* 2(1):5–9.

Torrance, G. (1998). Socio-historical overview: The development of the Canadian health system. In D. Coburn, C. D'Arcy, and G. M. Torrance (Eds.), *Health and Canadian society: Sociological perspectives,* third edition, pp. 3–22. Toronto: University of Toronto Press.

Travisano, R. V. (1981). Alternation and conversion as qualitatively different transformations. In G. P. Stone and H. A. Faberman (Eds.), *Social psychology through symbolic interaction,* pp. 237–248. New York: Wiley.

Trow, M. (1970). Comment on 'participant observation and interviewing: A comparison.' In W. J. Filstead, W. J. (Ed.), *Qualitative methodology: Firsthand involvement with the social world*, pp. 143–149. Chicago: Markham Publishing Company.

Trypuc, J. M. (1994). Women's health. In B. S. Bolaria and H. D. Dickinson (Eds.), *Health, illness, and health care in Canada*, second edition, pp. 260–275. Toronto: Harcourt Brace Canada.

Ullman, D. (1979). Holistic health as a model for personal and social change. *C/O: Journal of Alternative Human Services*, 5(2):9–12.

Veal, L. (1998). Complementary therapy and infertility: An Icelandic perspective. *Complementary Therapies in Nursing and Midwifery*, 4(1)3–6.

Vickers, A. (1993). *Complementary medicine and disability: Alternatives for people with disabling conditions*. London: Chapman and Hall.

Vickers, A. J. and Smith, C. (1997). Analysis of the evidence profile of the effectiveness of complementary therapies in asthma: A qualitative survey and systematic review. *Complementary Therapies in Medicine*, 5:202–209.

Vincent, C. A. and Furnham, A. (1997). The perceived efficacy of complementary and orthodox medicine: A replication. *Complementary Therapies in Medicine*, 5:85–89.

Vincent, C. and Furnham, A. (1996). Why do patients turn to alternative medicine? An empirical study. *British Journal of Clinical Psychology*, 35, 37–48.

Vincent, C. A. and Furnham, A. (1994). The perceived efficacy of complementary and orthodox medicine: Preliminary findings and the development of a questionnaire. *Complementary Therapies in Medicine*, 2:28–134.

Vincent, C. A., Furnham, A., and Willsmore, M. (1995). The perceived efficacy of complementary and orthodox medicine in complementary and general practice patients. *Health Education Research*, 10(4):394–405.

Walker, L. G. and Anderson, J. (1999). Testing complementary and alternative therapies within a research protocol. *European Journal of Cancer*, 35(11):1614–1618.

Wardwell, W. I. (1994). Alternative medicine in the United States. *Social Science and Medicine*, 38(8):1061–1068.

Wellman, B. (1995). Lay referral networks: Using conventional medicine and alternative therapies for low back pain. *Research in the Sociology of Health Care*, 12, 213–238.

White, A. and Ernst, E. (2001). The case for uncontrolled trials: A starting point for the evidence base for CAM. *Complementary Therapies in Medicine*, 9(2):61–132.

WHO. (2000). *World health report 2000*. World Health Organisation, publication on the Internet, viewed 15 January, 2001, http://www.who.int/whr/2000/en/report.html

Wolpe, P. R. (1990). The holistic heresy: Strategies of ideological challenge in the medical profession. *Social Science and Medicine*, 31(8):913–923.

Yamashita, H., Tsukayama, H., White, A. R., Tanno, Y., Sugishita, C., and Ernst, E. (2001). Systematic review of adverse events following acupuncture: the Japanese literature. *Complementary Therapies in Medicine*, 9(2):98–104.

Yates, P. M., Beadle, G., Clavarino, A., Najman, J. M., Thomson, D., Williams, G., Kenny, L., Roberts, S., Mason, B., and Schlect, D. (1993). Patients with terminal cancer who use alternative therapies: Their beliefs and practices. *Sociology of Health and Illness*, 15(2):199–216.

Ziegler, P. (1982). *The Black Death*. London: Penguin Books.

Zollman, C. and Vickers, A. (1999a). ABC of complementary medicine: Users and practitioners of complementary medicine. *British Medical Journal*, 319:836–838.

Zollman, C. and Vickers, A. (1999b). ABC of complementary medicine: Complementary medicine and the patient. *British Medical Journal*, 319:1486–1489.

Index